101 AMERICAN HERO Short Stories

Short Stories for Seniors

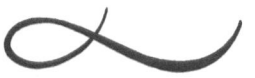

seniorality

101 American Hero Short Stories for Seniors -
Jamie Stonebridge, Sam Suncroft
Copyright © 2024
Seniorality / Everbreeze Media Oy

The stories presented in this book are based on factual research and historical records. While every effort has been made to ensure accuracy, the narratives contained herein are interpretations of real events and individuals.

Set in 16.5 pt EB Garamond

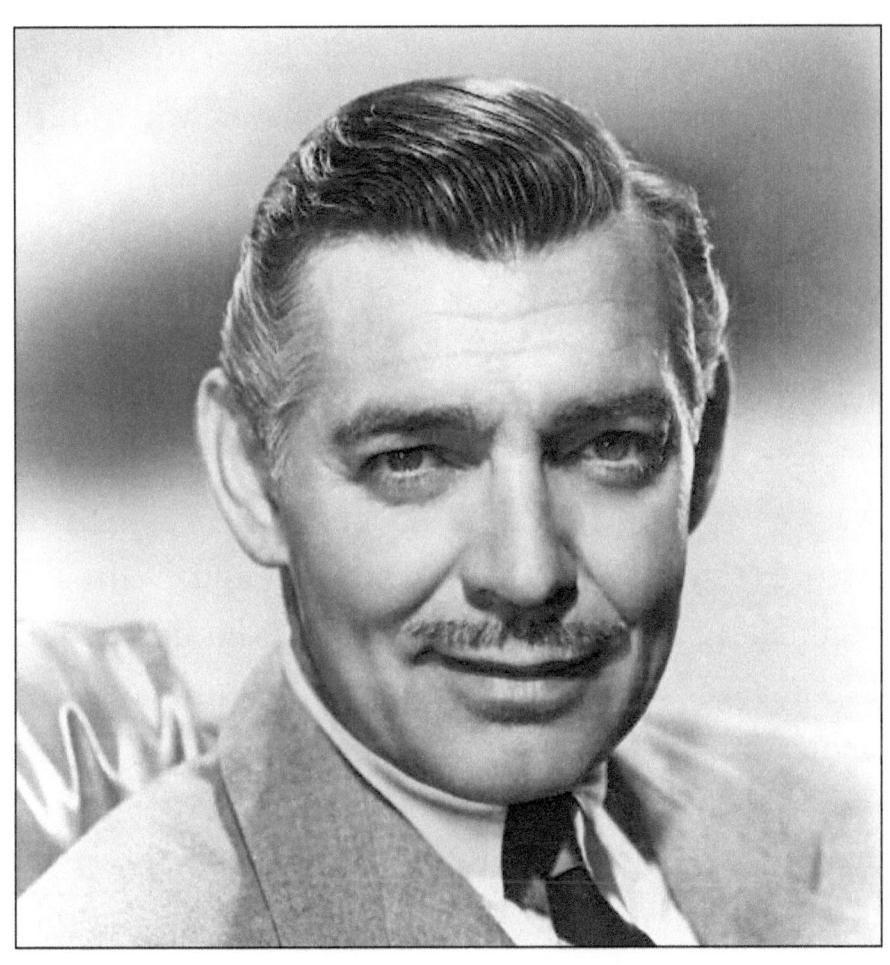

1. Clark Gable

Clark Gable, the iconic Hollywood actor known for his charisma and talent on the silver screen, also earned his place among the American heroes of World War II. Born on February 1, 1901, in Cadiz, Ohio, Gable's fame as a leading man in films such as "Gone with the Wind" and "It Happened One Night" cemented his status as a Hollywood legend. However, when duty called, Gable answered with bravery and selflessness, enlisting in the United States Army Air Forces (USAAF) in 1942.

Despite being in his forties, an age at which many men might have sought exemption from active duty, Gable was determined to serve his country in its time of need. He underwent rigorous training and eventually attained the rank of captain. But it was his decision to become an aerial gunner that truly showcased his dedication to the war effort.

Assigned to the 351st Bomb Group, Gable flew combat missions over Europe as a gunner, primarily aboard B-17 Flying Fortress bombers. These missions were perilous endeavors, fraught with danger as American crews faced fierce opposition from enemy fighters and anti-aircraft fire. Yet, Gable faced these dangers with the same courage and determination that marked his performances on screen.

His decision to serve in a combat role was not merely a publicity stunt or a token gesture of patriotism. Gable actively sought out the opportunity to put himself in harm's way alongside his fellow servicemen, embodying the spirit of sacrifice and solidarity that defined the Greatest Generation.

Throughout his time in the military, Gable not only demonstrated his bravery in combat but also forged lasting bonds with his fellow servicemen. He was respected and admired by his comrades, who saw in him a genuine commitment to their shared cause.

After the war, Gable returned to Hollywood, where he continued his illustrious career in film. However, his service in World War II remained a defining chapter in his life.

2. Jimmy Stewart

Jimmy Stewart, beloved actor and Hollywood icon, was not only a star on the silver screen but also a hero in the skies during World War II. Born on May 20, 1908, in Indiana, Pennsylvania, Stewart's career in acting catapulted him to fame with roles in classics like "It's a Wonderful Life" and "Mr. Smith Goes to Washington." Yet, when his country called, Stewart answered with bravery and dedication, enlisting in the United States Army Air Forces (USAAF) in 1941.

Commissioned as a second lieutenant, Stewart initially served as a flight instructor, leveraging his experience as a private pilot before the war. However, he yearned for a more active role in the conflict, and in 1943, he was assigned to the 445th Bombardment Group as a B-24 Liberator pilot.

Stewart's combat missions over Europe were harrowing experiences, marked by the constant threat of enemy fighters, flak, and mechanical failures. Despite the dangers, he flew with courage and determination, completing 20 combat missions with the 8th Air Force.

Stewart's service as a bomber pilot earned him several decorations, including the Distinguished Flying Cross, awarded for his valor and skill under fire. His leadership and bravery in the face of adversity inspired his crewmates and earned him the respect of his superiors.

Beyond his individual accomplishments, Stewart's humility and dedication to his fellow servicemen endeared him to all who served alongside him. He refused to seek special treatment or publicity for his actions, preferring to focus on his duties as a pilot and a leader.

3. Audie Murphy

Audie Murphy, hailed as one of the most decorated American combat soldiers of World War II, exemplified bravery, resilience, and heroism in the face of unimaginable adversity. Born on June 20, 1925, in Kingston, Texas, Murphy's upbringing was marked by hardship and poverty. However, when the United States entered World War II, Murphy saw an opportunity to serve his country and make a difference.

Enlisting in the United States Army at the age of 18, Murphy embarked on a journey that would test his courage and determination beyond measure. Despite his diminutive stature, standing at just 5 feet 5 inches tall, Murphy's tenacity and grit quickly earned him the respect of his comrades.

Assigned to the 15th Infantry Regiment, 3rd Infantry Division, Murphy saw action in some of the most intense and brutal battles of the European Theater. It was during the Allied invasion of Sicily that Murphy's valor first came to the fore, as he led his men with courage and determination in the face of overwhelming odds.

However, it was his actions in France that would cement Murphy's place in history as one of America's greatest war heroes. On January 26, 1945, near the village of Holtzwihr, Murphy's company came under heavy attack from German forces. Despite being outnumbered and outgunned, Murphy refused to back down, single-handedly taking out a German machine gun nest and leading a counterattack that repelled the enemy.

Murphy's extraordinary bravery that day earned him the Medal of Honor, the highest military decoration awarded for valor in action against an enemy force. His selfless actions saved countless lives and inspired his fellow soldiers to press on in the face of adversity.

After the war, Murphy's heroism continued to capture the imagination of the American public. He wrote a memoir detailing his experiences, which was later adapted into a successful Hollywood film, with Murphy himself starring as the lead.

4. Henry Fond

Henry Fonda, celebrated actor of stage and screen, also served his country with distinction during World War II as a member of the United States Navy. Born on May 16, 1905, in Grand Island, Nebraska, Fonda's career in Hollywood spanned decades and included iconic roles in films such as "The Grapes of Wrath" and "12 Angry Men."

In 1942, following the United States' entry into World War II, Fonda enlisted in the Navy, eager to contribute to the war effort. Despite being in his late thirties at the time, Fonda was determined to serve his country in whatever capacity he could.

During his service in the Navy, Fonda was assigned to the USS Satterlee, a destroyer escort ship that saw action in the Pacific Theater. As a member of the crew, Fonda played a vital role in escorting convoys, patrolling enemy waters, and providing support for Allied operations in the Pacific.

It was during his time in the Pacific Theater that Fonda's bravery and dedication to duty earned him the Bronze Star, a prestigious military decoration awarded for meritorious achievement or service in combat. Fonda's actions under fire exemplified the courage and resilience of the American servicemen fighting in some of the most challenging conditions of the war.

After the war, Fonda returned to Hollywood, where he continued his illustrious acting career, earning acclaim and accolades for his performances on stage and screen. Yet, his service in World War II remained a defining chapter in his life, shaping his character and instilling in him a deep sense of patriotism and duty.

Throughout his life, Fonda remained modest about his military service, preferring to focus on the contributions of his fellow servicemen rather than his own accomplishments. However, his bravery and selflessness in the face of danger served as an inspiration to all who knew him.

5. Lee Marvin

Lee Marvin, renowned actor and World War II veteran, exemplified courage and resilience both on and off the screen. Born on February 19, 1924, in New York City, Marvin's path to stardom was unconventional, shaped by his experiences as a Marine during World War II.

In 1942, at the age of 18, Marvin enlisted in the United States Marine Corps, eager to serve his country in its time of need. He was assigned to the 4th Marine Division and saw action in some of the bloodiest battles of the Pacific Theater, including the Battle of Saipan.

During the Battle of Saipan, which took place in June and July of 1944, Marvin's unit faced intense fighting against entrenched Japanese forces. Despite the ferocity of the enemy's resistance, Marvin displayed courage under fire, leading his fellow Marines with determination and bravery.

It was during the Battle of Saipan that Marvin was wounded in action, sustaining injuries that would earn him the Purple Heart, a prestigious military decoration awarded to those wounded or killed in combat. Despite his wounds, Marvin remained resolute in his commitment to his comrades and his country.

After recovering from his injuries, Marvin returned to the front lines and continued to serve with distinction until the end of the war. His experiences in combat left an indelible mark on him, shaping his outlook on life and instilling in him a deep sense of gratitude for the freedoms he had fought to defend.

After the war, Marvin embarked on a career in acting, where his rugged demeanor and commanding presence made him a natural fit for tough-guy roles in films such as "The Dirty Dozen" and "The Man Who Shot Liberty Valance." Yet, despite his success in Hollywood, Marvin never forgot his roots as a Marine and remained proud of his service to his country.

6. Robert Montgomery

Robert Montgomery, the distinguished actor and director, also served his country with valor and distinction during World War II. Born on May 21, 1904, in Beacon, New York, Montgomery's career in Hollywood spanned several decades and included roles in classics such as "Here Comes Mr. Jordan" and "Mr. and Mrs. Smith." Yet, when the call to arms sounded, Montgomery answered with bravery and dedication, enlisting in the United States Navy.

Commissioned as a lieutenant commander, Montgomery was assigned to the Pacific Theater, where he served as a naval officer aboard PT boats. These small, fast vessels played a crucial role in patrolling enemy waters, conducting reconnaissance missions, and engaging in hit-and-run attacks against Japanese forces.

Montgomery's leadership and courage under fire earned him the respect and admiration of his fellow sailors. He navigated treacherous waters and faced the constant threat of enemy attacks with unwavering resolve, exemplifying the bravery and determination of the American servicemen fighting in the Pacific.

As a naval officer aboard PT boats, Montgomery participated in numerous combat missions, including patrols along the coastlines of enemy-held territories and daring raids against Japanese shipping and shore installations. His actions played a vital role in the Allied campaign to secure control of the Pacific and defeat the Axis powers.

For his service during World War II, Montgomery was awarded the Navy Commendation Medal, recognizing his meritorious achievement and exceptional leadership in combat. His bravery and selflessness in the face of danger served as an inspiration to all who served alongside him.

7. Charles Durning

Born on February 28, 1923, in Highland Falls, New York, Charles Durning's journey to fame was preceded by his service in one of the most pivotal moments in history.

As a young man, Durning enlisted in the United States Army in 1944, eager to do his part in the war effort. He was assigned to the 1st Infantry Division, famously known as the "Big Red One," and took part in the Allied invasion of Normandy on June 6, 1944 — D-Day.

As the invasion force stormed the beaches of Omaha Beach under withering enemy fire, Durning displayed remarkable courage and determination. Despite the chaos and carnage around him, he pressed forward, aiding his fellow soldiers and helping to secure a foothold on the beachhead.

Throughout the course of the war, Durning saw action in numerous campaigns and battles across Europe. He fought in the Battle of the Bulge, one of the largest and bloodiest engagements of the war, and participated in the liberation of occupied territories as Allied forces pushed deeper into Nazi-occupied Europe.

Durning's bravery and resilience in the face of danger did not go unnoticed. He was wounded multiple times during his service, sustaining injuries that earned him the Purple Heart and other commendations for his valor and sacrifice.

After the war, Durning returned to civilian life, where he embarked on a successful acting career that spanned over five decades. He appeared in over 200 films, television shows, and stage productions, earning acclaim and accolades for his talent and versatility.

Charles Durning's courage and sacrifice on Omaha Beach and throughout the war serve as a testament to his bravery, resilience, and unwavering commitment to his country.

8. Paul Newman

Paul Newman, the legendary actor and philanthropist, answered the call to serve his country during World War II. Born on January 26, 1925, in Shaker Heights, Ohio, Newman's path to stardom was interrupted by his enlistment in the United States Navy.

In 1943, at the age of 18, Newman enlisted in the Navy and was trained as an aviation radioman and rear-seat gunner. He served in the Pacific Theater aboard aircraft carriers, where he flew as a rear-seat gunner in torpedo bombers.

Newman's duties as a rear-seat gunner were perilous, as he braved enemy fire and aerial combat to protect his aircraft and crewmates. His skill and bravery under fire earned him the respect and admiration of his fellow servicemen.

During his service in the Pacific, Newman witnessed firsthand the horrors of war and the sacrifices made by his comrades. He participated in numerous combat missions and patrols, facing the constant threat of enemy attack and the harsh realities of life at sea.

After the war, Newman returned to civilian life, where he pursued a career in acting that would ultimately make him one of the most beloved and respected actors of his generation. His talent and charisma endeared him to audiences around the world, earning him numerous awards and accolades throughout his illustrious career.

Despite his fame and success in Hollywood, Newman remained humble about his wartime experiences, often deflecting praise onto his fellow servicemen. However, his service in the Navy left an indelible mark on him, shaping his character and instilling in him a deep sense of duty and patriotism.

Throughout his life, Newman remained committed to giving back to his community and supporting charitable causes. He established the Newman's Own Foundation, which has donated over $550 million to charities around the world, and was actively involved in various philanthropic endeavors.

9. Kirk Douglas

Kirk Douglas, the iconic actor and producer, demonstrated his bravery and commitment to his country during World War II. Born on December 9, 1916, in Amsterdam, New York, Douglas's career in Hollywood would eventually span over six decades, earning him acclaim and recognition for his performances in classics such as "Spartacus" and "Paths of Glory."

In 1941, following the United States' entry into World War II, Douglas enlisted in the United States Navy. He served as a communications officer aboard the USS PC-1137, a submarine chaser tasked with escorting convoys and patrolling enemy waters.

During his service in the Navy, Douglas faced numerous dangers and challenges, including enemy attacks and the harsh conditions of life at sea. However, it was during a training exercise in 1944 that Douglas suffered severe injuries that would ultimately lead to his medical discharge from the Navy.

Despite the premature end to his military career, Douglas's service in the Navy left a lasting impact on him, shaping his character and instilling in him a deep sense of duty and patriotism. His experiences during the war would later inform his performances on screen, as he drew upon his own struggles and triumphs to bring authenticity to his roles.

After being discharged from the Navy, Douglas pursued his passion for acting, eventually finding success in Hollywood and becoming one of the most recognizable and respected actors of his generation. His talent and charisma captivated audiences around the world, earning him numerous awards and accolades throughout his career.

10. James Doohan

James Doohan, best known for his iconic role as Montgomery "Scotty" Scott in Star Trek, also had a remarkable military career during World War II. Born on March 3, 1920, in Vancouver, British Columbia, Canada, Doohan's path to fame was preceded by his service in the Royal Canadian Army.

In 1939, at the outbreak of World War II, Doohan enlisted in the Royal Canadian Army. He initially served as a member of the Royal Canadian Artillery, training as a field artillery crewman. However, his talents and skills would soon lead him to a different role within the military.

On June 6, 1944, Doohan participated in the Allied invasion of Normandy, famously known as D-Day. He landed on Juno Beach with the Royal Canadian Army's 3rd Infantry Division, where he faced intense fighting against entrenched German forces.

During the chaos of the D-Day landings, Doohan's bravery and determination shone through. Despite the overwhelming odds and the constant threat of enemy fire, he pressed forward, aiding his fellow soldiers and helping to secure a foothold on the beachhead.

It was during the Battle of Normandy that Doohan was wounded in action. Despite sustaining serious injuries, including being shot six times, Doohan miraculously survived, thanks in part to a silver cigarette case that deflected a bullet destined for his heart.

After recovering from his injuries, Doohan returned to the front lines and continued to serve with distinction until the end of the war. His bravery and sacrifice during World War II earned him several commendations, including the Distinguished Flying Cross for his actions in combat.

After the war, Doohan pursued a career in acting, where he would achieve fame and acclaim for his portrayal of Chief Engineer Montgomery "Scotty" Scott in Star Trek. Yet, despite his success in Hollywood, Doohan remained humble about his wartime experiences, often downplaying his own heroism and deflecting praise onto his fellow servicemen.

James Doohan's service in the Royal Canadian Army and his participation in the D-Day invasion, where he was wounded in action, stand as a testament to his bravery, resilience, and unwavering commitment to freedom.

11. Charlton Heston

Charlton Heston, served his country with honor and distinction during World War II. Born on October 4, 1923, in Evanston, Illinois, Heston's career in Hollywood would eventually span over six decades, earning him acclaim and recognition for his roles in classics such as "Ben-Hur" and "The Ten Commandments."

In 1944, at the height of World War II, Heston enlisted in the United States Army Air Forces. He underwent training as a radio operator and aerial gunner and was assigned to the 77th Bombardment Squadron, 28th Bombardment Group, flying aboard B-25 Mitchell bombers.

As a radio operator and aerial gunner, Heston played a vital role in the air war over Europe. He flew numerous combat missions, facing the constant threat of enemy fighters and anti-aircraft fire while providing support for Allied ground forces and conducting strategic bombing raids against Axis targets.

Heston's bravery and skill under fire earned him the respect and admiration of his fellow crewmates. Despite the dangers and hardships of aerial combat, he remained steadfast in his commitment to his country and his fellow servicemen.

After the war, Heston returned to civilian life, where he pursued his passion for acting and embarked on a successful career in Hollywood. His talent and charisma made him one of the most recognizable and respected actors of his generation, earning him numerous awards and accolades throughout his career.

12. James Stewart

James Stewart was born on May 20, 1908, in Indiana, Pennsylvania, Stewart's career in Hollywood would eventually span over five decades, earning him acclaim and recognition for his roles in classics such as "It's a Wonderful Life" and "Mr. Smith Goes to Washington."

In 1941, following the United States' entry into World War II, Stewart enlisted in the United States Army Air Forces (USAAF). Due to his prior experience as a pilot and his passion for aviation, Stewart was commissioned as a second lieutenant and underwent training as a pilot.

Stewart's skill and dedication quickly earned him the respect of his superiors, and he was soon assigned to the 445th Bombardment Group, where he flew bombing missions over Nazi-occupied Europe. As a bomber pilot, Stewart faced the constant threat of enemy fighters, flak, and adverse weather conditions while carrying out dangerous missions deep into enemy territory.

Despite the dangers and hardships of aerial combat, Stewart remained resolute in his commitment to his country and his fellow servicemen. He flew numerous combat missions, leading his crew with courage and determination in the face of adversity.

Stewart's bravery and leadership under fire earned him several commendations, including the Distinguished Flying Cross and the Air Medal with three oak leaf clusters, awarded for his valor and meritorious service in combat.

13. Gene Autry

Gene Autry, the iconic American singer, songwriter, actor, and businessman, served in the U.S. Army Air Forces during World War II. Born on September 29, 1907, in Tioga, Texas, Autry's career was marked not only by his immense success in entertainment but also by his service to his country during the war.

In 1942, Autry joined the Army Air Forces and was assigned to the Air Transport Command. As a part of this command, he flew cargo and transport missions primarily in the China-Burma-India (CBI) Theater of Operations.

Operating in challenging conditions, Autry and his fellow aircrew members navigated treacherous routes over rugged terrain and through hazardous weather to deliver essential supplies to Allied forces fighting in the remote regions of the CBI Theater. These missions were critical in supporting the war effort against Japanese forces in the region and sustaining Allied operations.

Autry's service in the Army Air Forces showcased his dedication, bravery, and commitment to the cause of freedom. Despite the dangers inherent in flying transport missions, he performed his duties with professionalism and courage.

After the war, Autry returned to his successful career in entertainment, where he continued to captivate audiences with his music, films, and television shows.

14. Neil Armstrong

Neil Armstrong, an American astronaut and aerospace engineer, made history on July 20, 1969, by becoming the first person to set foot on the Moon as part of NASA's Apollo 11 mission. Born on August 5, 1930, in Wapakoneta, Ohio, Armstrong's journey to the Moon was the culmination of years of dedication, training, and technological innovation.

As the commander of the Apollo 11 spacecraft, Armstrong, along with fellow astronauts Buzz Aldrin and Michael Collins, embarked on the historic mission to the lunar surface. After a journey of nearly 240,000 miles (386,000 kilometers) from Earth, the lunar module "Eagle" separated from the command module "Columbia" and descended towards the Moon's surface.

As millions of people around the world watched in awe, Armstrong piloted the lunar module with precision and skill, guiding it to a safe landing in the Sea of Tranquility. Upon stepping onto the lunar surface, he uttered the now-famous words: "That's one small step for [a] man, one giant leap for mankind."

Armstrong's historic moonwalk, which lasted just over two hours, marked a monumental achievement for humanity and a triumph of human ingenuity, determination, and exploration. It represented a giant leap forward in our understanding of the cosmos and our capabilities as a species.

After returning to Earth, Armstrong continued to make significant contributions to space exploration and science. He served as a professor of aerospace engineering at the University of Cincinnati and later as chairman of Computing Technologies for Aviation, Inc.

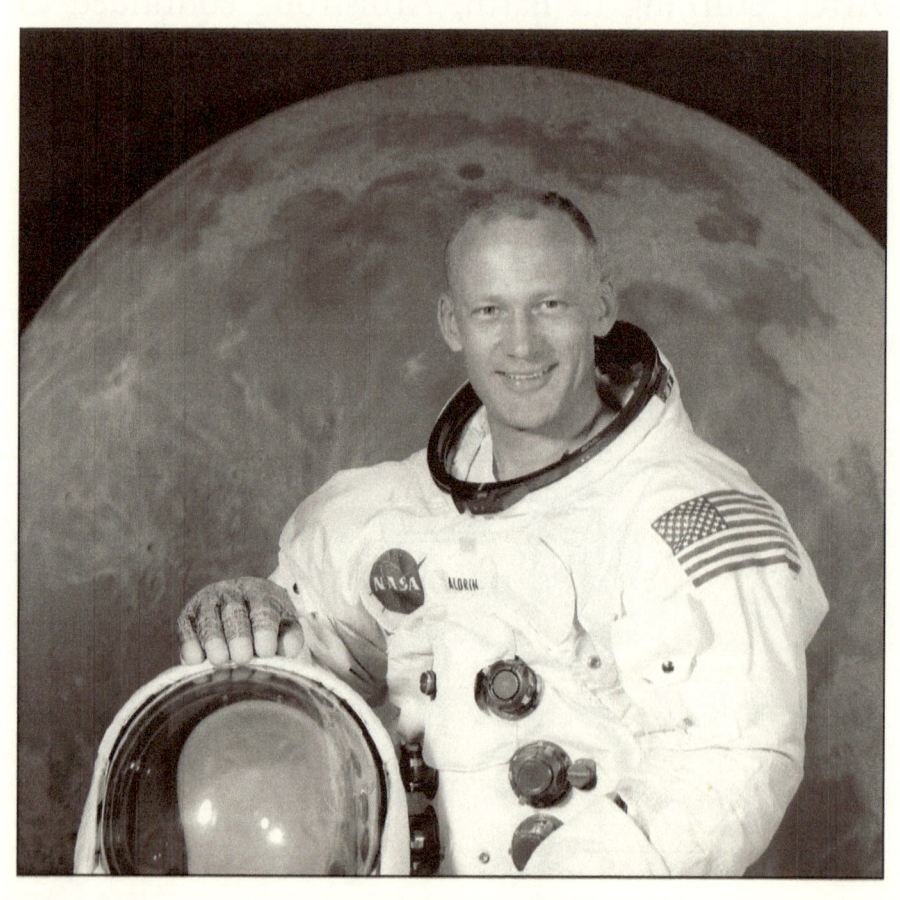

15. Buzz Aldrin

Buzz Aldrin, an American astronaut and engineer, made history on July 20, 1969, as part of NASA's Apollo 11 mission, becoming the second person to set foot on the Moon, shortly after Neil Armstrong. Born on January 20, 1930, in Glen Ridge, New Jersey, Aldrin's journey to the Moon was the culmination of years of training, dedication, and technological innovation.

As the Lunar Module Pilot of Apollo 11, Aldrin played a crucial role in the historic mission to the lunar surface. Alongside Neil Armstrong and Michael Collins, Aldrin traveled nearly 240,000 miles (386,000 kilometers) from Earth aboard the command module "Columbia" before descending to the lunar surface in the lunar module "Eagle."

After Armstrong's historic first step onto the Moon, Aldrin followed, becoming the second human to walk on its surface. As he descended the ladder of the lunar module, Aldrin described the momentous occasion as "magnificent desolation," capturing the stark beauty and solitude of the lunar landscape.

During their time on the lunar surface, Aldrin and Armstrong conducted scientific experiments, collected samples of lunar soil and rocks, and planted the American flag. Their historic moonwalks, which lasted just over two hours, marked a significant milestone in human history and represented a triumph of human ingenuity, courage, and exploration.

16. John Glenn

John Glenn, a pioneering American astronaut, made history on February 20, 1962, by becoming the first American to orbit the Earth as part of NASA's Mercury-Atlas 6 mission. Born on July 18, 1921, in Cambridge, Ohio, Glenn's journey to space was the culmination of years of dedication, training, and technological advancement.

As one of the original Mercury Seven astronauts selected by NASA, Glenn was chosen for his exceptional piloting skills, physical fitness, and personal qualities. On the day of the historic flight, Glenn boarded the Friendship 7 spacecraft and embarked on a journey that would captivate the world.

During his three-orbit flight around the Earth, Glenn faced numerous challenges and uncertainties, including concerns about the spacecraft's heat shield and reentry procedures. Despite these challenges, Glenn remained calm, focused, and determined to complete his mission.

As Friendship 7 streaked across the sky, Glenn provided valuable scientific data and observations, including insights into the effects of weightlessness on the human body and the behavior of spacecraft systems in orbit. His historic flight demonstrated America's capabilities in space and paved the way for future missions to explore the cosmos.

After his historic flight, Glenn continued to serve his country as a test pilot, astronaut, and United States Senator from Ohio. He returned to space in 1998 at the age of 77, becoming the oldest person to fly in space aboard the Space Shuttle Discovery's STS-95 mission.

17. Alan Shepard

Alan Shepard, an American astronaut and naval aviator, etched his name in history on May 5, 1961, by becoming the first American to journey into space as part of NASA's Mercury-Redstone 3 mission, also known as Freedom 7. Born on November 18, 1923, in East Derry, New Hampshire, Shepard's historic flight marked a significant milestone in the United States' space exploration efforts.

As a test pilot and experienced naval aviator, Shepard was chosen from a group of highly skilled astronauts to undertake the challenging task of piloting the Freedom 7 spacecraft into space. In the early morning hours of May 5, 1961, Shepard boarded the spacecraft atop a Redstone rocket at Cape Canaveral, Florida, and prepared for the historic flight.

During the 15-minute suborbital flight, Shepard experienced the thrill and excitement of space travel as he soared to an altitude of approximately 116 miles (187 kilometers) above the Earth's surface. Although the flight was brief compared to later space missions, it was a monumental achievement that demonstrated America's capabilities in space exploration.

After his historic flight, Shepard continued to serve NASA as an astronaut, eventually becoming the fifth person to walk on the Moon as commander of the

Apollo 14 mission in 1971. He later retired from NASA and pursued a career in business, but his legacy as the first American in space remains an enduring symbol of human achievement and exploration.

18. Sally Ride

Sally Ride, an American physicist and astronaut, made history on June 18, 1983, by becoming the first American woman to journey into space as part of NASA's STS-7 mission aboard the Space Shuttle Challenger. Born on May 26, 1951, in Los Angeles, California, Ride's historic flight marked a significant milestone in space exploration and inspired countless women and girls around the world.

As a graduate student in physics at Stanford University, Ride was selected as one of the first female astronauts in NASA's space program in 1978. Her selection as an astronaut was a testament to her exceptional intellect, determination, and passion for exploration.

On June 18, 1983, Ride blasted off into space aboard the Space Shuttle Challenger as a mission specialist, joining four other crew members on the STS-7 mission. During the six-day mission, Ride played a key role in deploying satellites, conducting scientific experiments, and operating the shuttle's robotic arm.

Ride's journey into space shattered gender barriers and demonstrated that women were just as capable as men of excelling in the demanding field of space exploration. Her courage, intelligence, and professionalism paved the way for future generations of female astronauts and inspired millions of people around the world.

19. Jim Lovell

Jim Lovell, an American astronaut and naval aviator, is best known as the commander of NASA's Apollo 13 mission, which encountered a life-threatening crisis while en route to the Moon in April 1970. Born on March 25, 1928, in Cleveland, Ohio, Lovell's career as an astronaut spanned over two decades and included four spaceflights.

Apollo 13 was intended to be the third mission to land humans on the lunar surface. Lovell, along with fellow astronauts Fred Haise and Jack Swigert, embarked on the mission aboard the Apollo spacecraft on April 11, 1970. However, two days into the mission, while the spacecraft was approximately 200,000 miles (320,000 kilometers) from Earth, an oxygen tank exploded, causing a catastrophic failure in the spacecraft's life support systems.

It was during this crisis that Lovell uttered the now-famous phrase, "Houston, we have a problem," informing mission control of the dire situation. The explosion forced the crew to abandon their plans to land on the Moon and instead focus on safely returning to Earth.

Through quick thinking, ingenuity, and cooperation between the astronauts and mission control, the crew of Apollo 13 successfully improvised solutions to critical problems, including carbon dioxide buildup, power shortages, and navigation challenges. Using the lunar module as a "lifeboat," the crew managed to return safely to Earth, splashing down in the Pacific Ocean on April 17, 1970.

Apollo 13 demonstrated the resilience, resourcefulness, and teamwork of NASA's astronauts and ground personnel. Lovell's calm leadership and quick decision-making under pressure played a crucial role in ensuring the crew's survival and safe return to Earth.

20. Eileen Collins

Eileen Collins, a retired American astronaut and United States Air Force colonel, made history as the first female Space Shuttle pilot and commander. Born on November 19, 1956, in Elmira, New York, Collins's pioneering career in space exploration spanned over two decades and included four spaceflights.

Collins joined NASA in 1990 and was selected as an astronaut candidate the following year. In 1995, she made history as the first female pilot of a Space Shuttle mission, serving as the pilot for STS-63 aboard the

Space Shuttle Discovery. During this mission, Collins and her crew conducted a rendezvous with the Russian space station Mir, marking the first time a Space Shuttle approached a space station from another country.

In 1999, Collins made history once again when she became the first female commander of a Space Shuttle mission, commanding STS-93 aboard the Space Shuttle Columbia. During this mission, Collins and her crew deployed the Chandra X-ray Observatory, a state-of-the-art telescope designed to observe X-rays from high-energy regions of the universe.

Collins's accomplishments as a pilot and commander paved the way for future generations of female astronauts and inspired women around the world to pursue careers in space exploration. Her leadership, professionalism, and dedication to the advancement of human spaceflight earned her widespread admiration and respect within the astronaut corps and the broader scientific community.

21. Gene Cernan

Gene Cernan, an American astronaut and naval aviator, made history as the last person to walk on the Moon during NASA's Apollo 17 mission in December 1972. Born on March 14, 1934, in Chicago, Illinois, Cernan's career as an astronaut spanned over a decade and included three spaceflights.

As the commander of Apollo 17, Cernan, along with astronauts Harrison Schmitt and Ronald Evans, embarked on a 12-day mission to the lunar surface. The Apollo 17 mission was the sixth and final lunar landing mission of NASA's Apollo program and remains the most recent manned mission to the Moon.

On December 11, 1972, Cernan and Schmitt descended to the lunar surface aboard the lunar module "Challenger" while Evans remained in lunar orbit aboard the command module "America." During their three days on the Moon, Cernan and Schmitt conducted scientific experiments, collected lunar samples, and explored the Taurus-Littrow Valley.

Cernan's historic moonwalk, which lasted just over 22 hours, marked the culmination of America's efforts to explore the Moon and represented a fitting conclusion to the Apollo program. As he prepared to depart the lunar surface, Cernan left behind a message on the surface of the Moon: "Here man completed his first explorations of the Moon, December 1972 A.D. May the spirit of peace in which we came be reflected in the lives of all mankind."

After returning to Earth, Cernan continued to serve NASA in various capacities, contributing to the development of the Space Shuttle program and other space exploration initiatives. He retired from NASA and the Navy in 1976.

22. Peggy Whitson

Peggy Whitson holds the record for the longest cumulative time spent in space by an American astronaut, with a total of 665 days spent in orbit over multiple missions. Born on February 9, 1960, in Mount Ayr, Iowa, Whitson's remarkable career in space exploration spanned over two decades and included three long-duration missions aboard the International Space Station (ISS).

Whitson's first spaceflight occurred in 2002 when she served as a flight engineer on Expedition 5 to the ISS. During her 184 days in space, Whitson conducted numerous scientific experiments and spacewalks, earning her widespread recognition for her contributions to research and exploration.

In 2007, Whitson returned to the ISS as the commander of Expedition 16, becoming the first female commander of the space station. During her 192-day mission, she oversaw the completion of critical construction and maintenance tasks and conducted groundbreaking scientific research in a variety of fields, including biology, physics, and medicine.

Whitson's third and final mission to the ISS took place in 2016 when she served as the commander of Expedition 50. During her 288-day mission, she continued to conduct research and experiments aimed at advancing our understanding of the effects of long-duration spaceflight on the human body and developing technologies to support future missions to deep space.

Throughout her career, Whitson demonstrated exceptional leadership, resilience, and dedication to the advancement of human space exploration. Her record-breaking achievements in space have earned her numerous awards and accolades, including the NASA Space Flight Medal and the Robert H. Goddard Memorial Trophy.

23. Chuck Yeager

Chuck Yeager, a legendary American test pilot and Air Force officer, made history on October 14, 1947, by becoming the first person to break the sound barrier in level flight. Born on February 13, 1923, in Myra, West Virginia, Yeager's groundbreaking achievement marked a pivotal moment in aviation history and paved the way for supersonic flight.

Flying the experimental Bell X-1 aircraft, nicknamed "Glamorous Glennis" after Yeager's wife, Yeager reached a speed of Mach 1.06, or approximately 700 miles per hour (1,127 kilometers per hour), at an altitude of 45,000 feet (13,700 meters) over the Mojave Desert in California. This historic flight shattered the long-standing belief that it was impossible for an aircraft to exceed the speed of sound without experiencing catastrophic aerodynamic effects.

Yeager's successful supersonic flight showed his exceptional piloting skills, courage, and determination. Despite facing numerous technical challenges and the inherent dangers of pushing the boundaries of aviation, Yeager remained calm and focused, guiding the X-1 through the sound barrier and into the annals of history.

Following his historic achievement, Yeager continued to push the boundaries of aviation as a test pilot, flying numerous experimental aircraft and breaking numerous speed and altitude records. He also served as a fighter pilot during World War II, where he distinguished himself in combat and earned the title of "ace" for shooting down at least five enemy aircraft in aerial combat.

24. Bob Hoover

Bob Hoover, an American aviation pioneer and legendary pilot, was renowned for his extraordinary aerobatic flying skills and his significant contributions to test flying. Born on January 24, 1922, in Nashville, Tennessee, Hoover's remarkable career spanned over seven decades and left an indelible mark on the world of aviation.

During World War II, Hoover served as a combat pilot in the United States Army Air Forces, flying Spitfire fighters with the 52nd Fighter Group. He was shot down over France, captured by the Germans, and spent 16 months as a prisoner of war. After the war, Hoover escaped from a German prison camp by stealing a German fighter plane and flying to safety in the Netherlands.

Following his wartime service, Hoover embarked on a career as a test pilot and aerobatic performer, dazzling audiences around the world with his breathtaking flying skills and precision maneuvers. He became known as the "pilot's pilot" for his mastery of the aircraft and his ability to push the limits of what was thought possible in the air.

One of Hoover's most famous feats was his demonstration of the "Hoover Nozzle," a technique he developed to showcase the remarkable performance capabilities of the North American P-51 Mustang fighter aircraft. This maneuver, which involved shutting off the engine in flight and performing a series of aerobatic maneuvers before restarting the engine, demonstrated Hoover's unmatched skill and confidence as a pilot.

In addition to his aerobatic performances, Hoover made significant contributions to test flying, working as a test pilot for North American Aviation and later for General Motors. He played a key role in the development and testing of numerous aircraft, including the F-86 Sabre, the F-100 Super Sabre, and the F-104 Starfighter.

Throughout his career, Hoover received numerous awards and accolades for his achievements in aviation, including the Distinguished Flying Cross, the Harmon Trophy, and induction into the National Aviation Hall of Fame.

25. Scott Crossfield

Scott Crossfield, an American test pilot and aeronautical engineer, achieved a historic milestone on November 20, 1953, by becoming the first person to fly at twice the speed of sound. Born on October 2, 1921, in Berkeley, California, Crossfield's pioneering flight marked a significant advancement in the field of aviation and helped pave the way for supersonic flight.

Crossfield achieved this historic feat while piloting the Douglas D-558-2 Skyrocket, an experimental research aircraft designed to explore high-speed flight regimes. The D-558-2 was equipped with a powerful turbojet engine and rocket motor, enabling it to reach speeds exceeding Mach 2, or twice the speed of sound.

On November 20, 1953, Crossfield climbed into the cockpit of the D-558-2 at Edwards Air Force Base in California and embarked on a daring test flight to push the boundaries of supersonic flight. During the flight, Crossfield accelerated the aircraft to a speed of Mach 2.005, or approximately 1,320 miles per hour (2,124 kilometers per hour), making him the first person to achieve sustained supersonic flight.

Crossfield's historic flight showed his exceptional piloting skills, courage, and dedication to advancing the field of aviation. His pioneering work in high-speed flight laid the groundwork for the development of supersonic aircraft such as the North American X-15 and the Concorde.

26. Jimmy Doolittle

Jimmy Doolittle, a pioneering American aviator and military leader, is best known for leading the famous "Doolittle Raid" during World War II. Born on December 14, 1896, in Alameda, California, Doolittle's career in aviation spanned several decades and included numerous accomplishments as a pilot, engineer, and military officer.

As tensions between the United States and Japan escalated in the early years of World War II, Doolittle, then a lieutenant colonel in the United States Army Air Forces (USAAF), proposed a daring plan to strike back at Japan with a surprise air raid on its home islands. The plan called for launching Army B-25 Mitchell bombers from an aircraft carrier, a feat that had never been attempted before.

On April 18, 1942, Doolittle led a squadron of 16 B-25 bombers from the USS Hornet aircraft carrier in the Western Pacific to launch a daring raid on Tokyo and other Japanese cities. The raid, although relatively modest in terms of damage inflicted, had a significant psychological impact, boosting American morale and demonstrating to the Japanese military that their homeland was vulnerable to attack.

After successfully executing the raid, Doolittle and his crew faced a perilous journey to escape capture by the Japanese. Several of the B-25s crash-landed or were forced to ditch at sea, and many crew members were captured or killed. Doolittle himself managed to evade capture and eventually made his way back to Allied territory.

For his leadership and valor during the Doolittle Raid, Doolittle was awarded the Medal of Honor, the United States' highest military decoration. He continued to serve with distinction throughout the war, commanding the Eighth Air Force in Europe and later contributing to the development of strategic bombing tactics.

27. Richard Bong

Richard Bong, an American fighter pilot, and flying ace, achieved legendary status during World War II as the top American ace of the conflict, credited with shooting down 40 Japanese aircraft. Born on September 24, 1920, in Poplar, Wisconsin, Bong's exceptional skill as a pilot and his remarkable success in aerial combat earned him widespread recognition and admiration.

Bong joined the United States Army Air Forces (USAAF) in 1941 and received flight training at various air bases across the United States. He quickly distinguished himself as a talented pilot, demonstrating exceptional flying ability and marksmanship during training exercises.

In 1942, Bong was deployed to the Pacific Theater of Operations, where he was assigned to the 49th Fighter Group, flying the Lockheed P-38 Lightning. Bong's first confirmed aerial victory came on December 27, 1942, when he shot down a Japanese Mitsubishi A6M Zero fighter near the island of Guadalcanal.

Over the next two years, Bong's tally of aerial victories continued to rise rapidly as he engaged in intense aerial combat against Japanese forces in the Pacific. He displayed extraordinary courage, skill, and determination in the face of formidable enemy opposition, earning him the nickname "Ace of Aces" and making him a hero among his fellow pilots.

Bong's most notable achievement came on December 17, 1944, when he surpassed Eddie Rickenbacker's World War I record of 26 aerial victories, becoming the top American ace of all time. By the end of the war, Bong's official tally stood at 40 confirmed aerial victories, making him the highest-scoring American pilot of World War II.

For his exceptional bravery and combat achievements, Bong was awarded the Medal of Honor, the United States' highest military decoration. He also received numerous other honors and awards for his valor in combat, including the Distinguished Service Cross, the Silver Star, and the Distinguished Flying Cross.

Tragically, Bong's illustrious career was cut short when he was killed in a flying accident on August 6, 1945, while testing a new aircraft in California.

28. Richard Winters

Richard Winters, was an American army officer, best known for his exemplary leadership as the commanding officer of Easy Company, 506th Parachute Infantry Regiment, 101st Airborne Division during World War II. Born on January 21, 1918, in New Holland, Pennsylvania, Winters played a pivotal role in some of the most significant battles of the European theater.

Winters' leadership and courage were immortalized in the book "Band of Brothers" by historian Stephen E. Ambrose and the subsequent HBO miniseries of the same name, which depicted the experiences of Easy Company throughout the war.

During World War II, Winters and Easy Company participated in some of the most crucial campaigns of the war, including the D-Day invasion of Normandy, the Battle of Carentan, Operation Market Garden, and the Battle of the Bulge. Winters' leadership under fire earned him the respect and admiration of his men, who regarded him as a fair and compassionate commander.

Winters' most famous act of leadership came during the Battle of Normandy on June 6, 1944. Despite being dropped several miles away from their intended drop zone and scattered in unfamiliar territory, Winters rallied his men and led a successful assault on a German battery at Brécourt Manor. Winters' decisive actions during this engagement earned him the Distinguished Service Cross, the United States' second-highest military decoration.

After the war, Winters returned to civilian life, eventually settling in Hershey, Pennsylvania, where he worked in a variety of roles, including as a businessman and public speaker. He remained humble about his wartime experiences, often deflecting praise onto his fellow soldiers and emphasizing the importance of teamwork and camaraderie.

29. Desmond Doss

Desmond Doss, an American army medic, and conscientious objector, exemplified extraordinary courage and selflessness during World War II, earning the Medal of Honor for his heroic actions in saving the lives of 75 wounded soldiers during the Battle of Okinawa. Born on February 7, 1919, in Lynchburg, Virginia, Doss's steadfast commitment to his beliefs and his unwavering bravery under fire made him a true American hero.

As a devout Seventh-day Adventist, Doss held strong religious convictions that prevented him from carrying a weapon or taking another person's life. Despite facing skepticism and opposition from his fellow soldiers and superiors, Doss remained resolute in his decision to serve as an unarmed combat medic, believing that he could save lives without compromising his beliefs.

During the Battle of Okinawa, one of the bloodiest conflicts of World War II, Doss's courage and compassion were put to the test. Amidst intense enemy fire and in the face of overwhelming odds, Doss repeatedly braved enemy fire to rescue wounded soldiers, lowering them down a sheer cliff face to safety below. Despite sustaining injuries himself, Doss refused to abandon his comrades, tirelessly tending to the wounded and risking his own life to save others.

Doss's extraordinary acts of heroism and selflessness earned him the Medal of Honor, the United States' highest military decoration. He became the first conscientious objector to receive the award for his actions on the battlefield, a testament to his unwavering commitment to his principles and his exceptional bravery under fire.

After the war, Doss returned to civilian life, where he continued to live out his values of compassion, service, and faith. He passed away on March 23, 2006, but his legacy as a true American hero lives on. Desmond Doss's remarkable story of courage, sacrifice, and conviction continues to inspire people around the world, serving as a powerful reminder of the extraordinary heights of human compassion and bravery, even in the midst of war.

30. David McCampbell

David McCampbell, a true American hero, distinguished himself as one of the most successful naval aviators of World War II. Born on January 16, 1910, in Bessemer, Alabama, McCampbell's journey to heroism began when he enlisted in the United States Naval Reserve in 1934. With a passion for aviation, he quickly rose through the ranks and earned his wings as a naval aviator.

McCampbell's combat prowess and leadership abilities were soon recognized, and he was assigned to serve aboard the USS Ranger, participating in operations in the Atlantic theater. However, it was in the Pacific theater where McCampbell would leave an indelible mark on history.

In 1943, McCampbell joined Air Group 15 aboard the USS Essex, a fleet carrier deployed to the Pacific to support Allied operations against Japan. As commander of Air Group 15, McCampbell led his squadron of F6F Hellcat fighters into some of the fiercest aerial battles of the war.

McCampbell's most significant moment came during the Battle of the Philippine Sea, also known as the "Great Marianas Turkey Shoot," in June 1944. Leading his squadron in defense of the American fleet, McCampbell's leadership and skill were put to the ultimate test against overwhelming Japanese forces.

In the span of just one day, McCampbell's extraordinary actions earned him a place in history. He single-handedly shot down nine Japanese aircraft, becoming the Navy's top ace of the Pacific theater and setting a record for the most aerial victories in a single mission. His exceptional performance during the battle earned him the Medal of Honor, the highest military decoration awarded by the United States.

Despite the accolades and recognition, McCampbell remained humble, attributing his success to the bravery and skill of his fellow pilots and the support of the sailors and crew aboard the USS Essex. Throughout the remainder of the war, McCampbell continued to lead his squadron with distinction, participating in numerous combat missions and earning additional awards and commendations for his bravery and leadership.

After the war, McCampbell continued to serve in the Navy, rising to the rank of rear admiral before retiring in 1964.

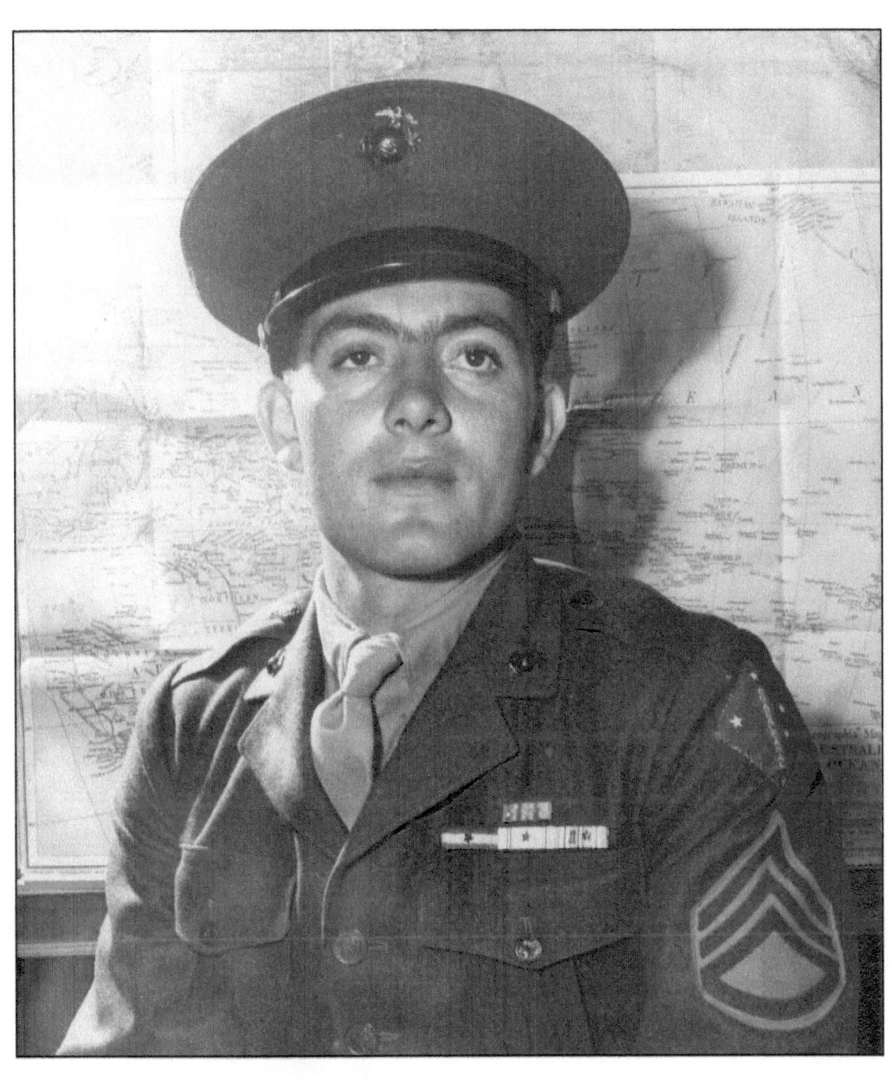

31. John Basilone

John Basilone, a United States Marine Corps gunnery sergeant, distinguished himself as a heroic and selfless leader during World War II, earning the Medal of Honor for his actions at the Battle of Guadalcanal.

Born on November 4, 1916, in Buffalo, New York, Basilone's bravery and valor in combat made him a legend among Marines and a symbol of courage and determination.

During the early stages of the Pacific campaign, Basilone served as a machine gun section leader with the 1st Battalion, 7th Marines, in the Solomon Islands. In October 1942, his unit came under heavy attack by Japanese forces during the Battle of Guadalcanal. Despite facing overwhelming odds and intense enemy fire, Basilone fearlessly manned his machine gun, delivering devastating firepower upon the enemy and providing crucial support to his fellow Marines.

Throughout the night-long battle, Basilone's leadership and courage inspired his men to hold their ground against repeated Japanese assaults. Despite sustaining multiple injuries, including shrapnel wounds and burns, Basilone continued to fight with unyielding determination, refusing to abandon his position until the enemy had been repelled.

Basilone's extraordinary actions during the Battle of Guadalcanal earned him the Medal of Honor, the United States' highest military decoration. His selfless sacrifice and unwavering devotion to duty exemplified the Marine Corps' core values of honor, courage, and commitment.

Following his heroic actions at Guadalcanal, Basilone returned to the United States and was hailed as a national hero. He participated in a war bond tour to raise funds for the war effort and was later commissioned as a second lieutenant. However, he chose to return to combat and was killed in action during the Battle of Iwo Jima on February 19, 1945.

32. James Garner

James Garner, the renowned American actor, was born on April 7, 1928, in Norman, Oklahoma. Garner served in the United States Army during the Korean War.

As a young man, Garner was drafted into the Army and deployed to Korea, where he served as a rifleman in the 5th Regimental Combat Team, a unit known for its fierce fighting in the Korean War. During his time in Korea, Garner saw action on the front lines and experienced the harsh realities of combat.

Garner's service in Korea was marked by acts of bravery and sacrifice, earning him two Purple Hearts for injuries sustained in battle. Despite facing the dangers of war, Garner remained steadfast in his commitment to his fellow soldiers and to the mission at hand.

After his honorable discharge from the Army, Garner pursued a career in acting, eventually achieving fame and success in Hollywood. He starred in numerous television shows and films, including the long-running series "Maverick" and "The Rockford Files," as well as iconic movies such as "The Great Escape" and "The Notebook."

33. Lewis Millett

Lewis Millett, a United States Army officer, distinguished himself as a fearless and courageous leader during the Korean War, earning the Medal of Honor for his heroic actions during the Battle of Hill 180. Born on December 15, 1920, in Mechanic Falls, Maine, Millett's bravery and valor in combat made him a legend among soldiers and a symbol of leadership and bravery.

During the Korean War, Millett served as a company commander in the 27th Infantry Regiment, 25th Infantry Division. On February 7, 1951, during the Battle of Hill 180 near Soam-Ni, South Korea, Millett's unit came under heavy attack by Chinese forces. Despite facing overwhelming odds and intense enemy fire, Millett fearlessly led his men in a bayonet charge up the hill, engaging the enemy in hand-to-hand combat and driving them from their positions.

Millett's decisive action and unwavering determination inspired his men to follow him into battle, and their courageous assault successfully secured the strategic position. His leadership under fire and his selfless devotion to duty earned him the Medal of Honor, the United States' highest military decoration.

Following his heroic actions at Hill 180, Millett continued to serve with distinction in the Army, eventually rising to the rank of colonel. He later served in the Vietnam War and held various command and staff positions throughout his military career.

34. Frederick W. Mausert III

Frederick W. Mausert III, a United States Marine Corps officer, demonstrated extraordinary bravery and leadership during the Vietnam War, earning the Medal of Honor for his heroic actions in leading his platoon in repelling multiple enemy assaults. Born on May 17, 1944, in Ridgewood, New Jersey, Mausert's courageous actions under fire made him a symbol of valor and selflessness.

During the Vietnam War, Mausert served as a first lieutenant in Company K, 3rd Battalion, 7th Marines, 1st Marine Division. On March 15, 1967, near the village of Que Son in Quang Nam Province, South Vietnam, Mausert's unit came under intense enemy fire from a well-fortified North Vietnamese position.

Despite being wounded early in the battle, Mausert refused medical attention and continued to lead his men in the defense of their position. Throughout the day, Mausert moved from one position to another, directing fire and rallying his men in the face of overwhelming odds.

As the enemy launched wave after wave of attacks, Mausert's leadership and courage never wavered. Despite being severely wounded again, he continued to lead his men with determination and resolve, inspiring them to fight on despite their fatigue and injuries.

Mausert's decisive actions and steadfast leadership ultimately turned the tide of the battle, enabling his platoon to repel the enemy assaults and secure their position. His extraordinary bravery and selflessness under fire earned him the Medal of Honor, the United States' highest military decoration.

After the war, Mausert returned to civilian life, where he continued to serve his country as a teacher and mentor to young people.

35. Montel Williams

Montel Williams, the accomplished American television personality, actor, and motivational speaker, served with distinction in the United States Marine Corps and participated in combat operations during the Vietnam War. Born on July 3, 1956, in Baltimore, Maryland, Williams' military service played a significant role in shaping his character and values.

After graduating from high school, Williams enlisted in the Marine Corps and completed basic training at Parris Island, South Carolina. He then underwent specialized training and was assigned to various units before ultimately deploying to Vietnam.

During his time in Vietnam, Williams served as a Marine Corps cryptologic technician, specializing in Morse code interception and analysis. He operated in dangerous and high-stress environments, providing crucial intelligence support to U.S. and allied forces during combat operations.

Williams' exemplary service in Vietnam earned him multiple commendations and awards, including the Navy Achievement Medal, the Navy Commendation Medal, and the Meritorious Service Medal. His dedication, professionalism, and courage under fire were recognized by his superiors and fellow Marines, and he was highly respected for his contributions to the mission.

After completing his military service, Williams transitioned to a career in television, where he achieved widespread fame and success as the host of "The Montel Williams Show" and as a guest on various talk shows and news programs. He has also been an advocate for veterans' issues, mental health awareness, and other social causes, using his platform to promote positive change and support for those in need.

36. Roy Benavidez

Roy Benavidez, a United States Army Special Forces soldier, displayed extraordinary heroism and selflessness during the Vietnam War, earning the

Medal of Honor for his actions in rescuing wounded soldiers during a fierce firefight. Born on August 5, 1935, in Lindenau, Texas, Benavidez's bravery and valor in combat made him a legend among soldiers and a symbol of courage and determination.

On May 2, 1968, while serving as a staff sergeant in the 5th Special Forces Group (Airborne), Benavidez was part of a 12-man Special Forces team operating near the border of Cambodia. The team was conducting a reconnaissance mission when they came under intense enemy fire from a much larger North Vietnamese force.

Despite being severely wounded in the initial volley of fire, Benavidez acted with incredible courage and disregard for his own safety. Ignoring his injuries, he bravely moved through the battlefield, administering first aid to wounded comrades and organizing their defense against the enemy.

Over the course of the six-hour battle, Benavidez repeatedly exposed himself to enemy fire as he evacuated wounded soldiers, retrieved critical supplies, and directed air support. Despite being shot multiple times and sustaining numerous injuries, including bayonet wounds and grenade fragments, Benavidez refused to be evacuated and continued to lead his men with unwavering determination.

Benavidez's heroic actions saved the lives of at least eight men and prevented the enemy from overrunning his team's position. His bravery and selflessness under fire earned him the Medal of Honor, the United States' highest military decoration.

After recovering from his injuries, Benavidez continued to serve in the Army, eventually rising to the rank of master sergeant. He remained active in veterans' affairs and served as a motivational speaker, inspiring others with his incredible story of courage and resilience.

37. Robert L. Howard

Robert L. Howard, a highly decorated United States Army Special Forces soldier, earned the Medal of Honor for his exceptional bravery and heroism in combat during the Vietnam War. Born on July 11,

1939, in Opelika, Alabama, Howard's remarkable courage and selflessness made him one of the most highly respected and admired soldiers in the history of the U.S. military.

Howard served multiple tours of duty in Vietnam as a member of the Special Forces, where he participated in numerous combat missions behind enemy lines. On December 30, 1968, during one such mission near the border of Cambodia, Howard's unit came under intense enemy fire from a much larger North Vietnamese force.

Despite being outnumbered and outgunned, Howard repeatedly exposed himself to enemy fire as he moved through the battlefield, rallying his men and directing their fire against the enemy. Throughout the course of the intense firefight, Howard single-handedly destroyed several enemy bunkers, rescued a wounded comrade, and led the successful evacuation of his unit from the battlefield.

Howard's extraordinary acts of bravery and selflessness under fire saved the lives of numerous comrades and prevented the enemy from overrunning his unit's position. His leadership and courage in the face of overwhelming odds earned him the Medal of Honor, the United States' highest military decoration.

In addition to the Medal of Honor, Howard was awarded the Distinguished Service Cross, the Silver Star, and eight Purple Hearts for wounds received in combat, making him one of the most highly decorated soldiers in American history.

38. Michael J. Novosel

Michael J. Novosel, a United States Army helicopter pilot, distinguished himself through extraordinary bravery and selflessness during the Vietnam War, earning the Medal of Honor for his heroic actions in rescuing wounded soldiers under heavy fire. Born on September 3, 1922, in Etna, Pennsylvania, Novosel's remarkable courage and dedication to his fellow soldiers made him a legend among aviators and a symbol of valor and compassion.

During the Vietnam War, Novosel served as a helicopter pilot with the 82nd Medical Detachment,

45th Medical Company, 68th Medical Group. On October 2, 1969, near Kien Tuong Province, South Vietnam, Novosel's helicopter was dispatched to evacuate wounded soldiers from a hotly contested battlefield.

Despite the intense enemy fire and adverse weather conditions, Novosel repeatedly flew his helicopter into the landing zone, braving enemy fire and risking his own life to evacuate wounded soldiers. Throughout the course of the mission, Novosel demonstrated exceptional skill and courage under fire, successfully evacuating a total of 29 wounded soldiers to safety.

Novosel's heroic actions saved the lives of numerous comrades and provided critical medical care to those in need. His selflessness and dedication to his fellow soldiers in the face of overwhelming odds earned him the Medal of Honor, the United States' highest military decoration.

In addition to the Medal of Honor, Novosel was awarded the Distinguished Flying Cross, the Bronze

Star Medal, and numerous other awards for his valor and service.

After retiring from the military, Novosel continued to serve his country as a civilian pilot and advocate for veterans' rights. He remained dedicated to honoring the sacrifices of his fellow soldiers and ensuring that their service and bravery were never forgotten.

39. Charles Liteky

Charles Liteky, a former United States Army chaplain, was awarded the Medal of Honor for his courageous actions in rescuing wounded soldiers under heavy fire during the Vietnam War. Born on February 14, 1931, in Washington, D.C., Liteky's extraordinary bravery and selflessness in the face of danger made him a hero among soldiers and a symbol of compassion and valor.

On December 6, 1967, near Phuoc-Lac, South Vietnam, Liteky's unit came under intense enemy fire while conducting a search and destroy mission. Despite being unarmed and exposed to enemy fire,

Liteky repeatedly braved the intense gunfire to evacuate wounded soldiers and administer medical aid.

Throughout the course of the battle, Liteky demonstrated exceptional courage and compassion, risking his own life to save the lives of his comrades. His unwavering dedication to his fellow soldiers in the face of overwhelming odds earned him the Medal of Honor, the United States' highest military decoration.

In addition to the Medal of Honor, Liteky was awarded the Purple Heart and numerous other awards for his valor and service.

After the war, Liteky became a peace activist and vocal critic of the Vietnam War. In 1986, he made headlines when he returned his Medal of Honor to then-President Ronald Reagan, citing his opposition to U.S. policies in Central America and his belief that the Medal of Honor should be a symbol of peace, not war.

40. Albert Einstein

Albert Einstein, one of the most influential scientists of the 20th century, was born on March 14, 1879, in Ulm, in the Kingdom of Württemberg in the German Empire. He is best known for his theory of relativity, which revolutionized our understanding of space, time, and gravity.

Einstein's early life was marked by academic curiosity and an independent spirit. He struggled in school, but his passion for physics and mathematics eventually led him to pursue advanced studies. In 1905, while working as a patent clerk in Bern, Switzerland, Einstein published four groundbreaking papers that laid the foundation for modern physics.

In 1915, Einstein published his theory of general relativity, which described gravity as the curvature of spacetime caused by the presence of mass and energy. This theory predicted the existence of phenomena such as black holes and gravitational waves, which were later confirmed by observations.

Einstein's contributions to physics earned him worldwide acclaim and numerous awards, including the Nobel Prize in Physics in 1921. However, he was also a vocal advocate for peace, civil rights, and social justice. He spoke out against war, militarism, and discrimination, and he was a prominent supporter of Zionism and the establishment of the state of Israel.

After fleeing Nazi Germany in 1933, Einstein settled in the United States, where he continued his scientific research and became a faculty member at the Institute for Advanced Study in Princeton, New Jersey. He remained active in academia and public life until his death on April 18, 1955.

41. Thomas Edison

Thomas Edison, often referred to as America's greatest inventor, was born on February 11, 1847, in Milan, Ohio, USA. He is renowned for his prolific contributions to various fields, particularly in electricity, telecommunications, and motion pictures.

Edison's most famous invention is the practical electric light bulb. He developed the first commercially viable and long-lasting incandescent light bulb in 1879. This innovation revolutionized indoor and outdoor lighting, transforming daily life by making it safer, more convenient, and extending productive hours.

In addition to the light bulb, Edison made significant contributions to the development of the electrical power system. He established the first electric power utility, the Edison Illuminating Company, and built the first power station in New York City in 1882, initiating the widespread adoption of electricity for lighting and other applications.

Edison's inventions were not limited to electricity. He held over 1,000 patents for various devices and processes, including the phonograph, which he invented in 1877, and the motion picture camera, which he developed in the late 19th century. His innovations in sound recording and motion pictures laid the foundation for the modern entertainment industry.

Throughout his life, Edison embodied the spirit of entrepreneurship and innovation. He founded numerous companies, including General Electric (GE), which became one of the largest and most influential corporations in the world. He also established research laboratories, such as the famous Edison Laboratory in Menlo Park, New Jersey, where he and his team conducted experiments and developed new technologies.

42. Jonas Salk

Jonas Salk, born on October 28, 1914, in New York City, was an American medical researcher and virologist best known for developing the first successful polio vaccine. His groundbreaking work saved countless lives and ushered in a new era in the fight against infectious diseases.

During the early 20th century, polio was a devastating disease that caused paralysis and death, especially among children. Salk became determined to find a way to prevent polio after witnessing its devastating effects firsthand as a medical student.

In the 1950s, Salk and his team developed a vaccine against polio using a killed virus. In 1955, after rigorous testing and clinical trials involving millions of children, the Salk vaccine was declared safe and effective. Its widespread distribution marked the beginning of the end of the polio epidemic in the United States and eventually worldwide.

Salk's vaccine was hailed as a medical miracle and a triumph of science. It not only saved countless lives but also led to the near-eradication of polio in many parts of the world. Salk became an international hero and a symbol of hope for millions of people affected by the disease.

Throughout his life, Salk remained dedicated to the pursuit of scientific knowledge and the betterment of humanity. He believed in the importance of collaboration and sharing scientific discoveries for the public good, famously stating, "The reward for work well done is the opportunity to do more."

43. Edwin Hubble

Edwin Hubble, born on November 20, 1889, in Marshfield, Missouri, was an American astronomer whose groundbreaking discoveries revolutionized our understanding of the universe. He is best known for his work in observational cosmology and for providing evidence that the universe is expanding.

After earning degrees in mathematics and astronomy, Hubble pursued a career in astronomy. In the 1920s, he made a series of remarkable observations using the newly built 100-inch telescope at Mount Wilson Observatory in California. Hubble's observations of distant galaxies revealed that they were receding from Earth, and the farther away a galaxy was, the faster it was moving away. This relationship, known as Hubble's Law, provided strong evidence for the expansion of the universe.

Hubble's discovery fundamentally changed our understanding of the cosmos. It supported the Big Bang theory, which posits that the universe began as a hot, dense state and has been expanding ever since.

Hubble's Law also laid the groundwork for the development of the modern field of cosmology, which seeks to understand the origin, evolution, and ultimate fate of the universe.

In addition to his work on the expansion of the universe, Hubble made many other important contributions to astronomy. He classified galaxies into different types based on their shapes and structures, a system known as the Hubble sequence.

Hubble's achievements earned him numerous awards and honors, including the Gold Medal of the Royal Astronomical Society and the Bruce Medal. The Hubble Space Telescope, launched in 1990, was named in his honor and has since provided astronomers with unparalleled views of the universe.

44. Benjamin Franklin

Benjamin Franklin, born on January 17, 1706, in Boston, Massachusetts, was one of the Founding Fathers of the United States and a polymath whose contributions spanned science, politics, diplomacy, and literature. He is perhaps best known for his role in drafting the Declaration of Independence and his service as an ambassador to France during the American Revolution, but his influence extended far beyond his political achievements.

Franklin was largely self-educated, having left school at an early age to apprentice as a printer. He became a successful businessman and publisher, founding the Pennsylvania Gazette newspaper and the Poor Richard's Almanack, which contained numerous aphorisms and proverbs that became widely quoted and admired.

In addition to his work as a printer and publisher, Franklin was a prolific inventor and scientist. He conducted experiments in electricity, famously demonstrating the nature of lightning and inventing the lightning rod to protect buildings from lightning strikes. His experiments with electricity led to important discoveries about the nature of electrical charge and conductivity.

Franklin was also a leading figure in the development of American civic life. He helped establish the first public library, fire department, and hospital in Philadelphia, and he played a key role in the founding of the University of Pennsylvania. He was a staunch advocate for free speech, religious tolerance, and representative government, and he served as a delegate to the Continental Congress and the Constitutional Convention.

In his later years, Franklin became increasingly involved in diplomacy and international affairs. He served as the first United States Minister to France from 1778 to 1785, where he played a crucial role in securing French support for the American Revolution and negotiating the Treaty of Paris, which ended the war and recognized American independence.

Benjamin Franklin's contributions to science, politics, and society have left an indelible mark on American history and culture. He embodied the spirit of the Enlightenment, advocating for reason, progress, and the pursuit of knowledge. His wit, wisdom, and ingenuity continue to inspire people around the world, and his legacy as a statesman, inventor, and thinker remains an enduring part of the American story.

45. Katherine Johnson

Katherine Johnson, born on August 26, 1918, in White Sulphur Springs, West Virginia, was an African American mathematician whose groundbreaking work at NASA played a crucial role in the success of the United States space program, particularly during the early years of manned spaceflight.

Johnson's exceptional mathematical skills were evident from a young age, and she graduated summa cum laude with degrees in mathematics and French from West Virginia State College. Despite facing racial and gender discrimination, she pursued a career in mathematics and teaching.

In 1953, Johnson joined the National Advisory Committee for Aeronautics (NACA), which later became NASA. She worked as a "human computer," performing complex calculations by hand for the agency's engineers and scientists.

Johnson's calculations were instrumental in numerous historic space missions, including the first manned spaceflight by an American, Alan Shepard's Mercury mission in 1961, and John Glenn's orbital flight aboard Friendship 7 in 1962. Her precise calculations helped ensure the safety and success of these missions, earning her the respect and admiration of her colleagues.

Despite the challenges of working in a male-dominated and racially segregated field, Johnson persevered and made significant contributions to the field of aerospace engineering.

In 2015, Johnson was awarded the Presidential Medal of Freedom, the highest civilian honor in the United States, for her contributions to space exploration and her pioneering achievements in mathematics. Her story gained widespread recognition with the release of the film "Hidden Figures" in 2016, which celebrated the contributions of Johnson and her fellow African American female mathematicians at NASA.

46. Rosa Parks

Rosa Parks, born on February 4, 1913, in Tuskegee, Alabama, was a civil rights activist whose courageous act of defiance helped ignite the Montgomery Bus Boycott and became a defining moment in the struggle for racial equality in the United States.

On December 1, 1955, Parks, a seamstress and NAACP (National Association for the Advancement of Colored People) member, refused to give up her seat to a white passenger on a segregated bus in Montgomery, Alabama. Her arrest for violating segregation laws sparked outrage and led to the launch of the Montgomery Bus Boycott, a coordinated protest against racial segregation on the city's buses.

The boycott, organized by civil rights leaders including Martin Luther King Jr., lasted for 381 days and marked the beginning of a new era in the civil rights movement. It demonstrated the power of nonviolent resistance and collective action in challenging racial injustice and galvanized support for the cause of civil rights nationwide.

Parks' act of resistance made her an iconic figure in the struggle for racial equality. She became known as the "mother of the civil rights movement" and inspired countless individuals to stand up against discrimination and oppression.

Throughout her life, Parks remained committed to the fight for justice and equality. She continued to work as a civil rights activist, advocating for desegregation, voter registration, and social justice. She received numerous awards and honors for her contributions to the civil rights movement, including the Presidential Medal of Freedom, the highest civilian honor in the United States.

47. Martin Luther King Jr.

Martin Luther King Jr., born on January 15, 1929, in Atlanta, Georgia, was a Baptist minister and civil rights leader who became the most prominent spokesperson and leader in the American civil rights movement from the mid-1950s until his assassination in 1968.

King emerged as a leader during the Montgomery Bus Boycott in 1955, sparked by Rosa Parks' refusal to give up her seat on a segregated bus. His leadership in the boycott demonstrated his commitment to nonviolent protest and civil disobedience as powerful tools for social change.

In 1957, King co-founded the Southern Christian Leadership Conference (SCLC), a nonviolent civil rights organization, and served as its first president. Through the SCLC, King organized and led numerous protests, marches, and demonstrations aimed at ending racial segregation and discrimination.

King's most famous speech, "I Have a Dream," delivered during the March on Washington for Jobs and Freedom in 1963, called for an end to racism and discrimination and envisioned a future of equality and justice for all Americans. The speech remains one of the most iconic and influential speeches in American history.

King's leadership and activism played a crucial role in the passage of landmark civil rights legislation, including the Civil Rights Act of 1964, which outlawed segregation in public places, and the Voting Rights Act of 1965, which aimed to eliminate racial barriers to voting.

Throughout his life, King faced numerous challenges and obstacles, including arrests, threats, and violence. However, he remained committed to his principles of nonviolence and love as the most potent weapons in the fight for justice and equality.

On April 4, 1968, King was assassinated in Memphis, Tennessee, while supporting a strike by African American sanitation workers. His death sparked riots and protests across the country and shocked the world.

Martin Luther King Jr.'s legacy as a champion of civil rights and social justice continues to inspire people around the world. His commitment to nonviolent resistance, his message of love and equality, and his vision of a beloved community built on justice and brotherhood remain as relevant today as they were during his lifetime.

48. Amelia Earhart

Amelia Earhart, born on July 24, 1897, in Atchison, Kansas, was an American aviator and pioneering pilot who became one of the most celebrated figures in aviation history. She was the first woman to fly solo across the Atlantic Ocean and set numerous other records during her career.

Earhart developed an early fascination with aviation and began taking flying lessons in 1921. In 1928, she became the first woman to fly across the Atlantic as part of a three-person crew, although she served primarily as a passenger. However, it was her solo transatlantic flight in 1932 that made her an international sensation. Earhart flew from Newfoundland to Ireland in just over 14 hours, becoming the first woman to complete the journey solo.

Throughout the 1930s, Earhart continued to set records and achieve milestones in aviation. She set speed and altitude records for female pilots, became the first person to fly solo from Hawaii to the mainland United States, and made numerous other groundbreaking flights.

In addition to her accomplishments as a pilot, Earhart was a tireless advocate for women's rights and an inspiration to millions of people around the world. She used her fame to promote gender equality and encourage women to pursue careers in aviation and other male-dominated fields.

Tragically, Earhart's career was cut short when she disappeared while attempting to circumnavigate the globe in 1937. Her plane vanished over the Pacific Ocean, and despite extensive search efforts, neither Earhart nor her aircraft were ever found. Her disappearance remains one of the greatest mysteries in the history of aviation.

49. Susan B. Anthony

Susan B. Anthony, born on February 15, 1820, in Adams, Massachusetts, was a prominent American suffragist, abolitionist, and social reformer who played a pivotal role in the fight for women's rights and equality.

Anthony devoted her life to advocating for women's suffrage, the right of women to vote and participate in the democratic process. She believed that women should have the same rights and opportunities as men and worked tirelessly to achieve this goal.

In 1869, Anthony and her close friend and collaborator Elizabeth Cady Stanton founded the National Woman Suffrage Association (NWSA), an organization dedicated to securing voting rights for women through an amendment to the U.S. Constitution. Anthony traveled across the country giving speeches, organizing rallies, and lobbying lawmakers to support women's suffrage.

Despite facing opposition and hostility from many quarters, Anthony never wavered in her commitment to the cause. She endured arrests, fines, and public ridicule for her activism but remained steadfast in her belief in the inherent equality of all people.

Anthony's efforts bore fruit when, in 1920, the Nineteenth Amendment to the U.S. Constitution was ratified, granting women the right to vote. Although Anthony did not live to see this victory—she passed away in 1906—her tireless advocacy laid the groundwork for the eventual success of the women's suffrage movement.

50. John Muir

John Muir, born on April 21, 1838, in Dunbar, Scotland, was a Scottish-American naturalist, author, and environmentalist who played a pivotal role in the conservation movement and the establishment of national parks in the United States.

Muir immigrated with his family to the United States in 1849, settling in Wisconsin. He developed a deep love and appreciation for the natural world at an early age, spending much of his time exploring the wilderness around his home.

In 1867, Muir embarked on a thousand-mile walk from Indiana to the Gulf of Mexico, during which he documented his observations of nature and cultivated his passion for conservation. This journey marked the beginning of his lifelong advocacy for the preservation of wild places.

Muir is perhaps best known for his role in the establishment of Yosemite National Park in California. His writings and advocacy were instrumental in convincing the U.S. Congress to pass legislation in 1890, granting Yosemite protected status as a national park, the third such park in the country.

Muir's efforts to protect Yosemite were part of a broader campaign to conserve and protect America's natural landscapes. He co-founded the Sierra Club in 1892, a conservation organization dedicated to preserving wilderness areas and promoting environmental stewardship. Muir served as the club's first president and played a central role in shaping its mission and goals.

Throughout his life, Muir wrote extensively about his experiences in nature and the importance of wilderness conservation. His books, essays, and articles helped popularize the idea of preserving natural landscapes for future generations and inspired countless people to explore and appreciate the beauty of the natural world.

51. Rachel Carson

Rachel Carson, born on May 27, 1907, in Springdale, Pennsylvania, was an American marine biologist, author, and conservationist whose groundbreaking book "Silent Spring" sparked the modern environmental movement and led to significant changes in pesticide regulation and environmental policy.

Carson developed an early passion for nature and science, which she pursued through her education and career. She earned a master's degree in zoology from Johns Hopkins University and began working as a marine biologist for the U.S. Bureau of Fisheries (later the U.S. Fish and Wildlife Service).

Carson's career as a writer began in the 1940s, when she published a series of articles and books about marine life and conservation. Her most famous work,

"Silent Spring," published in 1962, exposed the environmental and human health risks associated with the indiscriminate use of pesticides, particularly DDT.

"Silent Spring" warned of the dangers of pesticides to wildlife, particularly birds, and raised concerns about the potential long-term effects of pesticide contamination on ecosystems and human health. The book's title referred to the imagined silence that would result from the loss of birdsong due to pesticide poisoning.

Carson's powerful and meticulously researched book ignited a firestorm of controversy and debate. It sparked public outrage and prompted calls for greater regulation of pesticides and stronger environmental protections. "Silent Spring" is credited with helping to catalyze the modern environmental movement and leading to the banning of DDT and other harmful pesticides in the United States and around the world.

In addition to her environmental advocacy, Carson was also a passionate defender of wilderness and biodiversity. She believed in the intrinsic value of nature and the importance of preserving wild places for future generations.

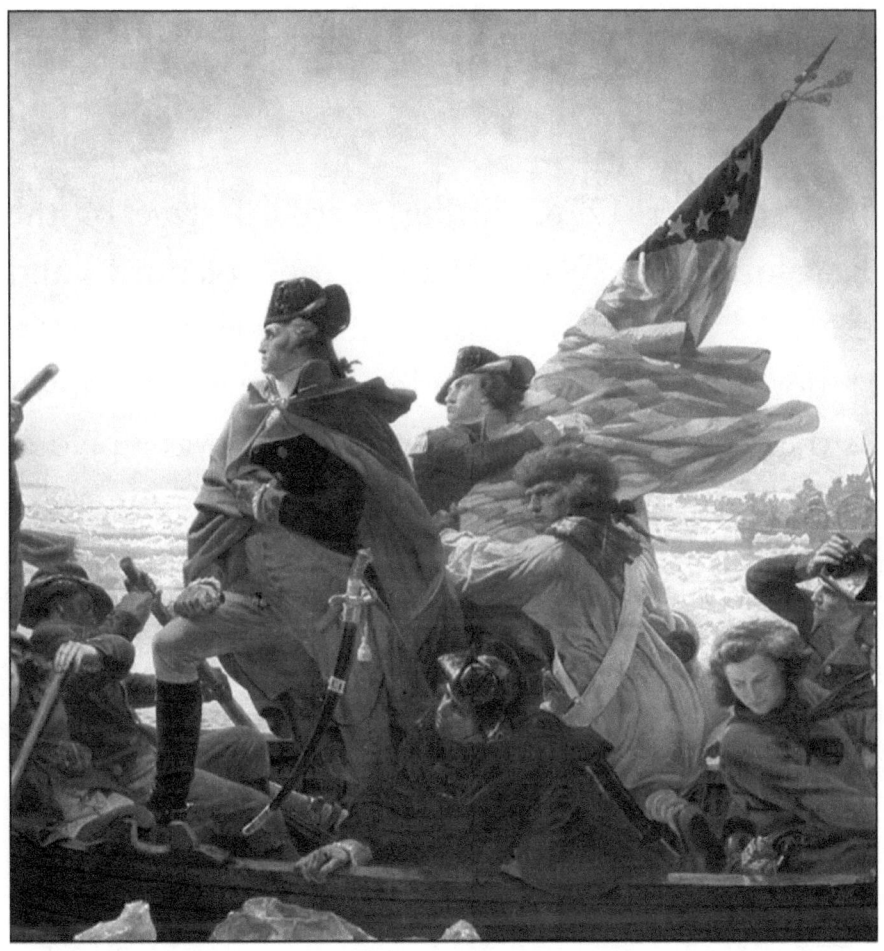

52. George Washington

George Washington, one of the Founding Fathers of the United States, was born on February 22, 1732, in

Westmoreland County, Virginia. He is best known for his role as the Commander-in-Chief of the Continental Army during the American Revolutionary War and as the first President of the United States.

In December 1776, during a crucial stage of the Revolutionary War, Washington planned and executed a daring surprise attack on Hessian forces stationed in Trenton, New Jersey. The event, known as the Crossing of the Delaware River, was a pivotal moment in the war and demonstrated Washington's leadership, strategic acumen, and determination to secure American independence.

Facing a series of defeats and setbacks earlier in the year, Washington recognized the need for a decisive victory to boost morale and rally support for the American cause. On the night of December 25-26, 1776, Washington and his troops crossed the icy Delaware River under treacherous conditions, braving freezing temperatures and harsh weather.

Despite the challenges of the crossing, Washington's forces successfully surprised the Hessian garrison at

Trenton in the early hours of December 26th. The American troops launched a swift and coordinated attack, capturing nearly 1,000 Hessian soldiers and dealing a significant blow to the British war effort.

The victory at Trenton bolstered American morale and reinvigorated the Revolutionary cause. It demonstrated Washington's leadership and strategic brilliance, proving that the Continental Army was capable of defeating the powerful British forces. The success of the Crossing of the Delaware River and the Battle of Trenton marked a turning point in the war and set the stage for future American victories.

53. Thomas Jefferson

Thomas Jefferson, born on April 13, 1743, in Shadwell, Virginia, was a key figure in the American Revolution and one of the Founding Fathers of the United States. He is best known as the primary author of the Declaration of Independence and the third President of the United States.

In June 1776, the Second Continental Congress appointed a committee to draft a formal statement of independence from Great Britain. Thomas Jefferson, a delegate from Virginia, was chosen to write the document, largely due to his eloquence and skill as a writer.

Jefferson worked diligently on the draft of the Declaration of Independence, drawing inspiration from Enlightenment ideals and the principles of natural rights and self-government. He famously wrote, "We hold these truths to be self-evident, that all men are created equal, that they are endowed by their Creator with certain unalienable Rights, that among these are Life, Liberty and the pursuit of Happiness."

On July 4, 1776, the Continental Congress adopted the Declaration of Independence, formally declaring the American colonies to be free and independent states. The document outlined the grievances against King George III and proclaimed the principles of liberty, equality, and self-determination.

The drafting of the Declaration of Independence marked a turning point in American history and solidified Thomas Jefferson's reputation as a champion of freedom and democracy. His eloquent words and visionary ideas helped inspire generations of Americans and set the stage for the establishment of a new nation founded on the principles of liberty and self-government.

In addition to his role in drafting the Declaration of Independence, Jefferson served as the third President of the United States from 1801 to 1809. During his presidency, he oversaw the Louisiana Purchase, which doubled the size of the United States, and championed principles of limited government, religious freedom, and individual rights.

Thomas Jefferson's contributions to American history and political thought are profound and enduring. His legacy as a statesman, philosopher, and visionary leader continues to inspire people around the world, reminding us of the enduring power of liberty, democracy, and the pursuit of happiness.

54. John Adams

John Adams, born on October 30, 1735, in Braintree, Massachusetts (now Quincy), was a Founding Father of the United States and a key figure in the American Revolution. He played a crucial role in advocating for independence from Great Britain and served on the committee responsible for drafting the Declaration of Independence.

Adams was a prominent lawyer and political leader in Massachusetts, known for his eloquence, intellect, and commitment to the cause of American independence. He became involved in colonial politics in the 1760s, opposing British policies such as the Stamp Act and the Townshend Acts that he viewed as infringements on American rights.

In 1774, Adams was elected as a delegate to the First Continental Congress, where he emerged as a leading voice for colonial rights and independence. He played a key role in drafting the Declaration of Rights and Grievances, which asserted the rights of the colonies and protested British policies.

Adams was also a delegate to the Second Continental Congress, where he continued to advocate for independence. He served on the committee responsible for drafting the Declaration of Independence, alongside Thomas Jefferson, Benjamin Franklin, Roger Sherman, and Robert Livingston. While Jefferson is credited as the primary author of the Declaration, Adams played a crucial role in shaping its content and securing its adoption by the Continental Congress on July 4, 1776.

After the Declaration of Independence was adopted, Adams continued to serve in various diplomatic and political roles during the Revolutionary War. He later served as the first Vice President of the United States under George Washington and was elected as the second President of the United States in 1796.

John Adams' contributions to the American Revolution and the founding of the United States were significant and enduring. His leadership, intellect, and dedication to the cause of independence helped to shape the course of American history and establish the principles of liberty, democracy, and self-government that continue to define the nation today. Adams' legacy as a Founding Father and statesman remains a source of inspiration and admiration for generations of Americans.

55. Paul Revere

Paul Revere, born on January 1, 1735, in Boston, Massachusetts, was a silversmith, engraver, and patriot who played a crucial role in the American Revolutionary War. He is best known for his "Midnight Ride" on April 18, 1775, during which he rode to warn of British troop movements prior to the battles of Lexington and Concord.

On the night of April 18, 1775, Revere and fellow patriot William Dawes were dispatched by Dr. Joseph Warren to alert colonial militia leaders of the impending arrival of British troops. Revere rode on horseback from Boston to Lexington, spreading the alarm along the way by knocking on doors and warning residents of the British advance.

Revere's famous ride, immortalized in Henry Wadsworth Longfellow's poem "Paul Revere's Ride," played a critical role in alerting the colonial militia and enabling them to prepare for the British attack. Thanks in part to Revere's warning, colonial forces were able to confront the British troops at Lexington and Concord, marking the beginning of the American Revolutionary War.

Although Revere's ride was only one part of a larger network of riders and messengers spreading the alarm throughout Massachusetts, his name became synonymous with the spirit of American independence and resistance to British tyranny. He became a hero of the Revolution and a symbol of courage, patriotism, and defiance in the face of oppression.

In addition to his famous Midnight Ride, Paul Revere was also known for his work as a skilled silversmith and engraver. He created numerous works of art and functional objects, including intricate silverware, teapots, and engravings, which are highly prized today for their craftsmanship and historical significance.

56. Patrick Henry

Patrick Henry, born on May 29, 1736, in Hanover County, Virginia, was a prominent American orator, lawyer, and Founding Father who played a key role in the movement for American independence. He is best known for his passionate speeches advocating for liberty and self-government, including his famous "Give me liberty, or give me death!" speech delivered at the Virginia Convention in 1775.

On March 23, 1775, Patrick Henry delivered his stirring speech at St. John's Church in Richmond, Virginia, during the Second Virginia Convention. In his speech, Henry passionately urged his fellow Virginians to take up arms against British tyranny and fight for independence. He famously declared:

"Is life so dear, or peace so sweet, as to be purchased at the price of chains and slavery? Forbid it, Almighty God! I know not what course others may take; but as for me, give me liberty, or give me death!"

Henry's powerful words galvanized support for the American cause and inspired many to join the fight for independence. His speech captured the spirit of the Revolution and became a rallying cry for patriots throughout the colonies.

In addition to his oratorical skills, Patrick Henry was also a skilled lawyer and politician. He served as the first governor of Virginia after independence and played a leading role in the movement to ratify the U.S. Constitution. He was a staunch advocate for states' rights and a vocal opponent of centralized government power.

Patrick Henry's contributions to the American Revolution and the founding of the United States were significant and enduring. His passionate advocacy for liberty and self-government helped to inspire the American people to rise up against British oppression and establish a new nation based on the principles of freedom and democracy. Henry's legacy as a patriot and orator continues to be remembered and celebrated today, reminding us of the power of words to inspire action and change.

57. John Paul Jones

John Paul Jones, born on July 6, 1747, in Arbigland, Scotland, was a naval commander and American Revolutionary War hero known for his daring exploits and bold leadership. He is best remembered for his famous declaration, "I have not yet begun to fight!" during his command of the USS Bonhomme Richard in its victorious engagement with the HMS Serapis in 1779.

In September 1779, during the American Revolutionary War, John Paul Jones commanded the USS Bonhomme Richard, a converted merchant ship, as part of a squadron tasked with disrupting British shipping in the North Sea. On September 23, 1779, the squadron encountered a British convoy escorted by the HMS Serapis and HMS Countess of Scarborough off the coast of Flamborough Head, England.

In the ensuing battle, the Bonhomme Richard engaged the Serapis in a fierce and brutal fight. Despite being outgunned and outmanned, Jones and his crew fought valiantly, enduring heavy casualties and sustaining severe damage to their ship. As the battle raged on, the Serapis captain reportedly called out to Jones, asking if he had surrendered. Jones's defiant response became legendary:

"I have not yet begun to fight!"

Undeterred by the odds stacked against him, Jones continued to press the attack, eventually forcing the surrender of the Serapis after a brutal hand-to-hand struggle. The victory was a remarkable achievement for Jones and a significant morale boost for the American cause.

John Paul Jones's victory over the Serapis cemented his reputation as one of the greatest naval commanders of the Revolutionary War and earned him international acclaim. His daring raid on British shipping and his fearless leadership exemplified the spirit of American independence and defiance in the face of overwhelming odds.

In addition to his famous victory aboard the Bonhomme Richard, John Paul Jones went on to serve with distinction in the Continental Navy and the Russian Navy, earning a reputation as a skilled strategist and tactician.

58. Francis Marion

Francis Marion, born on February 26, 1732, in Berkeley County, South Carolina, was a military officer and patriot who played a key role in the American Revolutionary War. He earned the nickname "Swamp Fox" for his skillful leadership of guerrilla warfare tactics against the British in South Carolina.

Marion's military career began during the French and Indian War, where he served as a lieutenant in the South Carolina militia. He gained valuable experience in wilderness warfare and tactics, which would later prove instrumental in his leadership during the Revolutionary War.

As the conflict with Britain escalated in the South, Marion emerged as a prominent figure in the patriot cause. He organized and led a group of irregular militia fighters known as Marion's Brigade, who operated in the swamps and forests of South Carolina.

Marion's guerrilla warfare tactics were highly effective against the British forces. He and his men conducted raids and ambushes against British supply lines, outposts, and patrols, harassing and disrupting enemy operations. Marion's intimate knowledge of the terrain and his ability to move quickly and strike unexpectedly earned him a fearsome reputation among the British and made him a hero to the American cause.

One of Marion's most famous exploits was the Battle of Black Mingo Creek in 1780, where his forces successfully ambushed and defeated a larger British detachment. This victory boosted patriot morale and helped to secure Marion's legacy as a skilled military leader.

Throughout the Revolutionary War, Francis Marion continued to lead his militia fighters in hit-and-run attacks against the British, contributing to the overall success of the American war effort in the South. His tactics and leadership played a significant role in wearing down British forces and ultimately contributing to the American victory.

After the war, Marion served in various political roles in South Carolina, including as a state senator and a member of the Continental Congress. He died on February 27, 1795.

59. John Hancock

John Hancock, born on January 23, 1737, in Braintree, Massachusetts (now Quincy), was a prominent American statesman and Founding Father who played a leading role in the American Revolution. He is best known as the President of the Second Continental Congress and the first signer of the Declaration of Independence.

As President of the Second Continental Congress, Hancock presided over the deliberations that led to the adoption of the Declaration of Independence on July 4, 1776. When it came time to sign the document, Hancock's signature stood out for its size and boldness, making his name synonymous with a person's signature.

Legend has it that Hancock's large signature was intended as a defiant gesture toward the British authorities, symbolizing his commitment to the cause of American independence. Although there is no definitive evidence to support this claim, Hancock's bold signature has become an iconic symbol of American defiance and patriotism.

In addition to his role in the Continental Congress, Hancock played a significant role in Massachusetts politics and was a key figure in the early stages of the American Revolution. He was a member of the Massachusetts Provincial Congress and served as president of the Massachusetts Provincial Congress.

Hancock's leadership and support for the patriot cause made him a target of British authorities, who viewed him as a dangerous rebel. In April 1775, British troops were ordered to arrest Hancock and fellow patriot Samuel Adams in Lexington, Massachusetts, sparking the first shots of the

Revolutionary War at the Battles of Lexington and Concord.

After the war, John Hancock continued to serve in various political roles, including as the first Governor of Massachusetts and a member of the Continental Congress. He died on October 8, 1793, leaving behind a legacy as one of the most prominent and influential figures of the American Revolution.

60. George Rogers Clark

George Rogers Clark, born on November 19, 1752, near Charlottesville, Virginia, was an American military officer and frontiersman who played a crucial role in securing the western frontier during the American Revolutionary War. He is best known for leading the capture of British-held forts in the Illinois country, including the capture of Fort Vincennes in 1779.

In the early years of the Revolutionary War, the British controlled a series of forts in the Ohio Valley and the Illinois country, which they used as bases to support their Native American allies and launch raids against American settlements on the western frontier. Recognizing the strategic importance of these forts, George Rogers Clark conceived a daring plan to capture them and secure the western frontier for the American cause.

In the winter of 1778-1779, Clark led an expedition of frontier militia and Kentucky volunteers on a grueling march through the wilderness to attack the British-held forts in the Illinois country. Despite facing harsh conditions and logistical challenges, Clark and his men successfully captured several key forts, including Fort Kaskaskia and Fort Cahokia, without firing a shot.

The most dramatic and celebrated victory of Clark's campaign came with the capture of Fort Vincennes (present-day Vincennes, Indiana) in February 1779. The fort was heavily fortified and defended by a sizable British garrison, but Clark's bold tactics and strategic maneuvering caught the British by surprise. After a daring nighttime march through flooded terrain, Clark and his men launched a surprise attack on the fort, overwhelming the defenders and forcing them to surrender.

The capture of Fort Vincennes was a significant victory for the American cause. It secured American control over the Illinois country and helped to weaken British influence in the western frontier. Clark's campaign also disrupted British plans to launch raids against American settlements and Native American allies in the region.

61. Daniel Morgan

Daniel Morgan, born on July 6, 1736, in Hunterdon County, New Jersey, was a Continental Army general and a hero of the American Revolutionary War. He is best known for his leadership at the Battle of Cowpens, a pivotal engagement that marked a turning point in the Southern campaign.

In January 1781, during the Southern theater of the Revolutionary War, Daniel Morgan commanded American forces at the Battle of Cowpens in South Carolina. Facing a superior British force led by

Lieutenant Colonel Banastre Tarleton, Morgan devised a brilliant strategy that exploited the terrain and the strengths of his troops.

Morgan positioned his men in three lines: skilled marksmen and militia in the front, followed by Continental regulars, and a reserve force in the rear. He also ordered his cavalry to feign retreat, drawing the British forces into a trap.

As the British advanced, Morgan's troops unleashed a devastating volley of musket fire, decimating the enemy ranks. The American militia then fell back to the second line, where they were reinforced by the Continentals. The British, believing they had the advantage, pressed forward, only to be met with another withering volley from Morgan's men.

In a desperate attempt to break the American lines, Tarleton ordered a cavalry charge, but it was repulsed by disciplined fire from the American infantry. Meanwhile, the American cavalry, having regrouped after their feigned retreat, launched a devastating counterattack on the British flank.

The combined effect of Morgan's strategy and the valor of his troops resulted in a resounding American victory at Cowpens. The British suffered heavy casualties, including the capture of over 600 men, while the Americans suffered relatively few losses.

The Battle of Cowpens was a decisive victory for the American cause in the Southern campaign. It boosted morale among American troops, weakened British control over the region, and set the stage for further American successes leading to the eventual surrender of British forces at Yorktown later that year.

62. Sybil Ludington

Sybil Ludington, born on April 5, 1761, in Fredericksburg, New York, was a teenage girl who played a heroic role in the American Revolutionary War. She is best known for her courageous midnight ride to warn of a British raid on Danbury, Connecticut, earning her the nickname "the female Paul Revere."

On the night of April 26, 1777, sixteen-year-old Sybil Ludington received word that British troops were marching towards Danbury, Connecticut, intending to raid the town and destroy its military supplies. With her father, Colonel Henry Ludington, away on duty as a militia officer, Sybil took it upon herself to warn the local militia and muster reinforcements.

Riding alone through the dark and rainy night, Sybil covered over 40 miles, much farther than Paul Revere's famous ride, to spread the alarm and summon the militia to defend Danbury. She rode through rugged terrain, ford rivers, and navigate wooded trails, facing the danger of encountering British soldiers or hostile Native American tribes along the way.

By dawn, Sybil had successfully alerted the militia and gathered a force of over 400 men to defend Danbury. Although the British troops succeeded in their raid and destroyed much of the town, the American forces were able to engage them in skirmishes and hinder their progress, ultimately forcing them to retreat.

Sybil Ludington's courageous ride and quick thinking helped to mobilize the local militia and mitigate the damage caused by the British raid on Danbury. Her bravery and determination in the face of danger made her a symbol of the contributions of ordinary Americans, including women and young people, to the Revolutionary cause.

63. Samuel Adams

Samuel Adams, born on September 27, 1722, in Boston, Massachusetts, was a Founding Father of the United States and a key figure in the American Revolution. He is best known for his role as a political agitator and organizer of colonial resistance to British rule.

In the years leading up to the American Revolution, Samuel Adams emerged as a leading voice of opposition to British policies in the American colonies. He was a staunch advocate for colonial rights and played a central role in organizing protests against British taxation policies, particularly the Stamp Act and the Townshend Acts.

In 1765, Adams was one of the founders of the Sons of Liberty, a secret organization dedicated to resisting British tyranny and promoting colonial rights and liberties. The Sons of Liberty organized protests, boycotts, and acts of civil disobedience to oppose British taxation and other oppressive measures.

One of the most famous acts of resistance organized by Samuel Adams and the Sons of Liberty was the Boston Tea Party in 1773. In response to the Tea Act, which granted the British East India Company a monopoly on tea imports to the colonies, Adams and his fellow patriots disguised themselves as Native Americans and boarded British ships in Boston Harbor, dumping over 300 chests of tea into the water in protest.

Adams was also instrumental in organizing colonial resistance to the Intolerable Acts, a series of punitive measures imposed by the British government in response to the Boston Tea Party. He helped to convene the First Continental Congress in 1774, where colonial delegates gathered to coordinate their response to British oppression and assert their rights as British subjects.

Throughout the Revolutionary War, Samuel Adams continued to play a leading role in the patriot cause, serving in the Continental Congress and advocating for independence. He signed the Declaration of Independence in 1776 and later served as governor of Massachusetts.

64. Douglas MacArthur

Douglas MacArthur, born on January 26, 1880, in Little Rock, Arkansas, was a prominent American military leader who played a key role in several major conflicts of the 20th century, including World War I, World War II, and the Korean War. He is best known for his leadership as a general who commanded Allied forces in the Pacific Theater during World War II.

During World War II, MacArthur commanded Allied forces in the Southwest Pacific Theater, where he played a crucial role in the defeat of Japanese forces. He developed and executed a strategy of "island hopping," bypassing heavily fortified Japanese positions and seizing strategically important islands to advance closer to Japan.

One of MacArthur's most significant achievements was the liberation of the Philippines from Japanese occupation. After the fall of the Philippines in 1942, MacArthur famously vowed, "I shall return." In 1944, he fulfilled that promise, leading Allied forces in the successful recapture of the Philippines in a series of hard-fought battles, including the Battle of Leyte Gulf.

MacArthur's leadership in the Pacific Theater earned him widespread acclaim and established him as one of the most respected military commanders of his time. His strategic vision, combined with his bold and decisive leadership style, contributed to the eventual defeat of Japan and the end of World War II.

After the war, MacArthur played a prominent role in the occupation and reconstruction of Japan, serving as Supreme Commander for the Allied Powers. He oversaw the democratization and rebuilding of Japanese society, implementing far-reaching reforms aimed at transforming Japan into a peaceful and democratic nation.

MacArthur's career was not without controversy, particularly his handling of the Korean War. As commander of United Nations forces in Korea, he pursued a bold but controversial strategy, including the daring amphibious landing at Inchon. However, his insistence on advancing to the Yalu River, which bordered China, ultimately led to a Chinese intervention and a protracted stalemate.

65. Dwight D. Eisenhower

Dwight D. Eisenhower, born on October 14, 1890, in Denison, Texas, was a prominent American military leader and statesman who played a pivotal role in World War II and later served as the 34th President of the United States. He is best known for his leadership as Supreme Allied Commander in Europe during the D-Day invasion and for his efforts to promote peace and prosperity during his presidency.

During World War II, Eisenhower rose through the ranks of the U.S. Army to become one of the most respected and trusted military leaders of his time. In 1942, he was appointed Supreme Commander of the Allied Expeditionary Force, tasked with planning and executing the invasion of Nazi-occupied Europe.

On June 6, 1944, Eisenhower oversaw the largest amphibious assault in history, known as Operation Overlord or the D-Day invasion. Under his command, Allied forces landed on the beaches of Normandy, France, in a daring and meticulously coordinated operation that marked the beginning of the end for Nazi Germany.

Eisenhower's leadership and strategic acumen were instrumental in the success of the D-Day invasion, which paved the way for the liberation of Western Europe from Nazi tyranny. His calm demeanor, decisive decision-making, and ability to inspire confidence in his troops earned him the admiration and respect of Allied commanders and soldiers alike.

After the war, Eisenhower served as Military Governor of the American Zone in Germany and then as Chief of Staff of the U.S. Army before retiring from active duty in 1948. In 1952, he was elected as the 34th President of the United States, serving two terms from 1953 to 1961.

As President, Eisenhower pursued a moderate and pragmatic agenda, focusing on domestic issues such as infrastructure development, civil rights, and the economy. He also championed a policy of containment in the Cold War, seeking to prevent the spread of communism while avoiding direct military confrontation with the Soviet Union.

Eisenhower's presidency was marked by relative peace and prosperity, earning him the nickname "Ike" and widespread popularity among the American people.

66. George S. Patton

George S. Patton, born on November 11, 1885, in San Gabriel, California, was a highly influential and controversial American military leader known for his bold and aggressive leadership style. He played a key role in World War II as a commander of armored units in North Africa and Europe.

Patton was a career Army officer who distinguished himself early in his military career for his leadership and tactical acumen. He gained recognition for his role in the development and effective use of armored warfare tactics, advocating for the importance of tanks and mechanized infantry in modern warfare.

During World War II, Patton commanded the U.S. Seventh Army during the Allied invasion of North Africa in Operation Torch in 1942. His leadership and aggressive tactics played a crucial role in the success of the campaign, helping to defeat Axis forces in North Africa and secure control of the region.

Patton's most famous campaign came in 1944 when he commanded the U.S. Third Army during the Allied invasion of Normandy and subsequent operations in Western Europe. He led his troops in a series of rapid and audacious advances across France, earning a reputation as one of the most effective battlefield commanders of the war.

Patton's leadership of the Third Army was characterized by his emphasis on speed, mobility, and aggressive offensive action. He pushed his troops to their limits, often leading from the front and inspiring them with his fearless and determined demeanor.

Despite his military successes, Patton was a controversial figure known for his outspoken and sometimes abrasive personality. He was known for his colorful language, strict discipline, and occasionally controversial remarks, which sometimes landed him in hot water with his superiors.

George S. Patton died on December 21, 1945, from injuries sustained in a car accident in Germany.

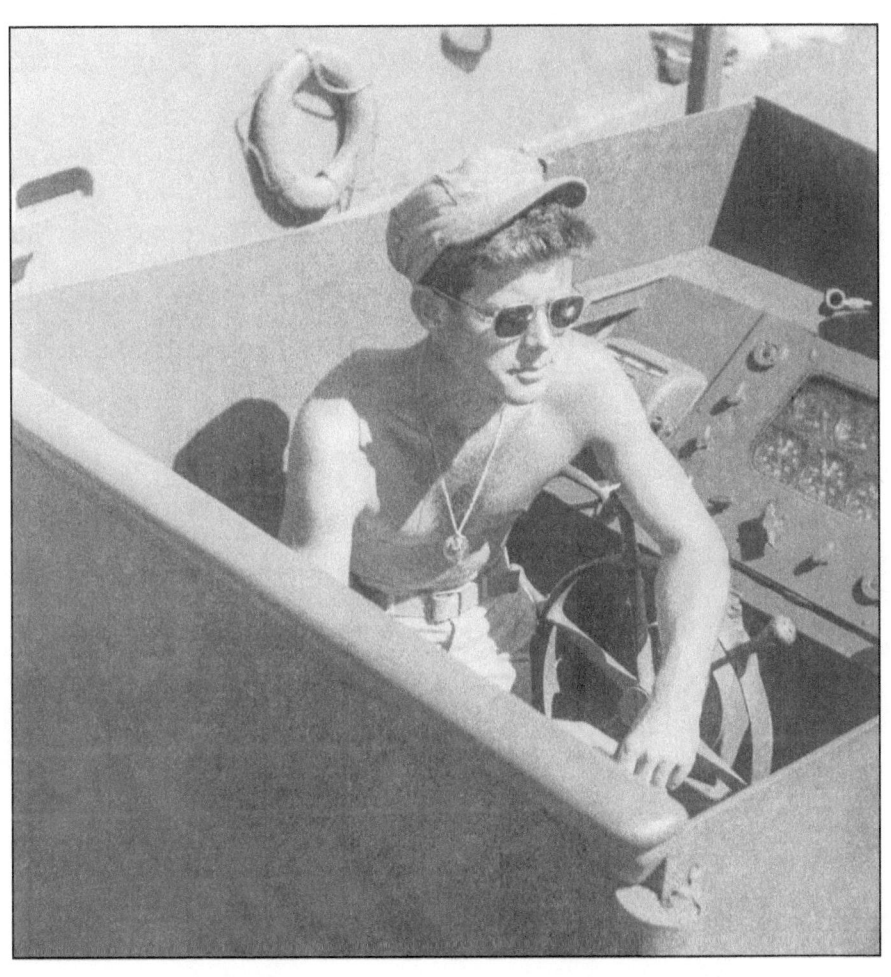

67. John F. Kennedy

John F. Kennedy, born on May 29, 1917, in Brookline, Massachusetts, was a prominent American statesman who served as the 35th President of the United States. Before his political career, Kennedy served as a Navy officer during World War II, commanding a patrol torpedo boat in the Pacific Theater.

In 1941, shortly after the United States entered World War II, John F. Kennedy enlisted in the Navy. He was assigned to the Office of Naval Intelligence in Washington, D.C., and later requested a transfer to sea duty.

In 1943, Kennedy was appointed as the commanding officer of PT-109, a patrol torpedo boat assigned to the Solomon Islands in the South Pacific. On the night of August 1, 1943, PT-109 was rammed and sunk by a Japanese destroyer during a night patrol. Kennedy and his crew swam to a nearby island, where they awaited rescue.

Kennedy's leadership and resourcefulness during the ordeal earned him praise and admiration from his crew and superiors. He helped to rescue injured crew members and led them to safety, despite suffering from back injuries himself.

After being rescued by a group of Solomon Islanders, Kennedy continued to serve in the Navy until 1945, when he was honorably discharged due to his wartime injuries. He was awarded the Navy and Marine Corps Medal and the Purple Heart for his actions during the sinking of PT-109.

Following his military service, John F. Kennedy entered politics, serving as a congressman from Massachusetts and later as a senator before being elected President of the United States in 1960. As president, Kennedy faced numerous challenges, including the Cuban Missile Crisis, the Bay of Pigs invasion, and the Civil Rights Movement.

Despite his abbreviated presidency, John F. Kennedy left a lasting legacy as a charismatic leader who inspired a generation of Americans. His tragic assassination in 1963 shocked the nation and led to an outpouring of grief around the world.

68. Richard Winters

Richard Winters, born on January 21, 1918, in New Holland, Pennsylvania, was a highly respected Army officer who played a pivotal role in World War II as the commanding officer of Easy Company, 2nd Battalion, 506th Parachute Infantry Regiment, 101st Airborne Division. He led Easy Company during the D-Day invasion and the Battle of the Bulge, among other crucial engagements.

Winters joined the U.S. Army in 1941 and volunteered for the paratroopers, undergoing rigorous training to become a member of the elite 101st Airborne Division. He quickly rose through the ranks due to his leadership abilities and was eventually promoted to the rank of captain and given command of Easy Company.

On June 6, 1944, Winters and Easy Company parachuted into Normandy as part of the D-Day invasion, landing behind enemy lines in the early hours of the morning. Despite being scattered and disoriented, Winters rallied his men and led them in capturing key objectives, including the strategic causeway bridges near the town of Carentan.

Winters' leadership during the chaotic and intense fighting of D-Day earned him widespread admiration and respect among his men and his superiors. His calm demeanor under fire and his ability to make quick, decisive decisions were credited with saving many lives and ensuring the success of the mission.

Winters continued to lead Easy Company through the grueling campaigns of the European Theater, including the airborne assault on Holland during Operation Market Garden and the bitter winter fighting in the Ardennes during the Battle of the Bulge.

One of Winters' most famous actions came during the Battle of the Bulge when he led a successful assault on the German-held town of Foy. Despite being vastly outnumbered and facing heavy enemy fire, Winters and his men captured the town, inflicting heavy casualties on the enemy and earning Winters the Distinguished Service Cross for his bravery and leadership.

After the war, Richard Winters returned to civilian life, eventually settling in Hershey, Pennsylvania, where he worked as a businessman. He remained humble about his wartime exploits and shunned the spotlight, but his leadership and heroism during

World War II were immortalized in Stephen E. Ambrose's book "Band of Brothers" and the subsequent HBO miniseries of the same name.

69. Richard Bong

Richard Bong, born on September 24, 1920, in Superior, Wisconsin, was a highly decorated Army Air Forces pilot and the top American ace of World War II. He is credited with shooting down 40 Japanese aircraft, making him one of the most successful fighter pilots in U.S. military history.

Bong enlisted in the U.S. Army Air Forces in 1941 and trained as a fighter pilot. He was assigned to the Pacific Theater of Operations, where he flew the Lockheed P-38 Lightning, a twin-engine fighter aircraft known for its speed and firepower.

Bong quickly distinguished himself as a skilled and aggressive pilot, racking up an impressive tally of aerial victories against Japanese aircraft. His tactics and marksmanship earned him the respect of his fellow pilots and the admiration of his superiors.

Bong's most famous exploit came on December 27, 1944, when he shot down his 40th enemy aircraft, surpassing the previous record held by Major Thomas McGuire. Bong's record of 40 aerial victories made him the top American ace of World War II and earned him numerous awards and decorations, including the Medal of Honor, the Distinguished Service Cross, and the Silver Star.

Despite his extraordinary combat record, Bong remained modest and unassuming, preferring to let his actions speak for themselves. He was known for his humility and his dedication to his fellow pilots, often sharing his knowledge and experience to help them improve their skills.

Tragically, Bong's life was cut short when he was killed in a crash while testing a new jet aircraft on August 6, 1945, just days before the end of the war. He was posthumously promoted to the rank of major and awarded the Medal of Honor for his extraordinary heroism and devotion to duty.

70. Benjamin Lewis Salomon

Benjamin Lewis Salomon, born on September 1, 1914, in Milwaukee, Wisconsin, was a dentist and a commissioned officer in the United States Army Dental Corps during World War II. He is best known for his heroic actions as a combat medic during the Battle of Saipan, for which he posthumously received the Medal of Honor.

Salomon volunteered for military service in 1940 and was commissioned as a first lieutenant in the Dental Corps. Despite being a non-combatant due to his role as a dentist, Salomon underwent additional training as a surgeon to better serve his fellow soldiers in combat situations.

In June 1944, during the Battle of Saipan in the Pacific Theater, Salomon found himself thrust into a front-line combat role when Japanese forces launched a fierce assault on his field hospital. Despite being wounded himself, Salomon refused to evacuate and instead remained behind to treat wounded soldiers and defend his position.

As the enemy closed in, Salomon continued to treat the wounded and defend his makeshift hospital with rifle and machine gun fire. He personally killed dozens of enemy soldiers and inflicted heavy casualties on the attacking forces.

In the final hours of the battle, Salomon was fatally wounded while manning a machine gun to cover the evacuation of wounded patients. Despite his injuries, he continued to provide covering fire until he was overwhelmed by enemy forces and killed.

For his extraordinary bravery and selflessness in the face of overwhelming odds, Benjamin Salomon was posthumously awarded the Medal of Honor, the highest military decoration awarded by the United States government. His citation praised his "conspicuous gallantry and intrepidity at the risk of his life above and beyond the call of duty."

71. John William Finn

John William Finn, born on July 24, 1909, in Los Angeles, California, was a United States Navy officer who received the Medal of Honor for his heroic actions during the attack on Pearl Harbor on December 7, 1941. Finn's courageous defense of his base, despite being wounded multiple times, earned him the distinction of being the first Medal of Honor recipient of World War II.

As the Japanese launched their surprise attack on Pearl Harbor, then-Chief Aviation Ordnanceman Finn was stationed at Naval Air Station Kaneohe Bay on Oahu, Hawaii. When the attack began, Finn immediately sprang into action, manning a .50 caliber machine gun mounted on an exposed platform despite the intense enemy fire.

Despite sustaining numerous wounds from shrapnel and bullets, Finn remained at his post, courageously firing his machine gun at the attacking Japanese aircraft. He continued to fire until he was ordered to seek medical attention, refusing to leave his position until he was physically unable to continue.

Finn's actions during the attack on Pearl Harbor were credited with downing at least one enemy aircraft and inflicting significant damage on others. His relentless defense of his base and his selfless bravery in the face of overwhelming odds inspired his fellow servicemen and earned him the admiration of his superiors.

For his extraordinary heroism and devotion to duty, John Finn was awarded the Medal of Honor by President Franklin D. Roosevelt in recognition of his "conspicuous devotion to duty, extraordinary courage, and complete disregard for his own life." He became the first Medal of Honor recipient of World War II, setting a high standard of courage and selflessness for others to emulate.

After the attack on Pearl Harbor, Finn continued to serve in the Navy, eventually rising to the rank of lieutenant.

John William Finn passed away on May 27, 2010, at the age of 100, leaving behind a legacy of courage, honor, and selfless service.

72. Vernon Joseph Baker

Vernon Joseph Baker, born on December 17, 1919, in Cheyenne, Wyoming, was an African American soldier who posthumously received the Medal of Honor for his extraordinary bravery and leadership during combat in Italy during World War II. He became one of the few black recipients of the award for his actions on the battlefield.

Baker served in the segregated U.S. Army during World War II and was assigned to the 370th Infantry Regiment, a unit composed primarily of African American soldiers. Despite facing discrimination and prejudice, Baker proved himself to be a capable and courageous soldier, rising to the rank of first lieutenant.

On April 5-6, 1945, during the Italian Campaign, Baker's unit was assigned the task of attacking and securing a series of heavily fortified enemy positions near Viareggio, Italy. Despite being outnumbered and facing intense enemy fire, Baker led his men with exceptional bravery and determination.

During the attack, Baker single-handedly destroyed several enemy positions, personally killing numerous enemy soldiers and knocking out machine gun nests and artillery emplacements. Despite being wounded multiple times, he continued to lead his men forward, inspiring them with his fearless leadership and unwavering courage.

Baker's actions during the battle were instrumental in the success of his unit's mission, and his bravery under fire saved the lives of many of his fellow soldiers.

In 1997, more than fifty years after the end of World War II, Vernon Baker's valor and sacrifice were finally recognized when he was awarded the Medal of Honor by President Bill Clinton in a ceremony at the White House. He became one of the few African American soldiers to receive the nation's highest military decoration for valor during World War II.

73. Elaine Danforth Harmon

Elaine Danforth Harmon, born on November 23, 1919, in Rockville, Maryland, was a pioneering aviator who served as a Women Airforce Service Pilot (WASP) during World War II. She later became a passionate advocate for the recognition of the WASP as veterans, leading to their posthumous award of the Congressional Gold Medal.

As a WASP, Elaine Harmon was part of a group of civilian female pilots who flew military aircraft during World War II, ferrying planes from factories to military bases, towing targets for live anti-aircraft artillery practice, and performing other non-combat flight duties. Despite facing discrimination and skepticism from some male pilots and military officials, the WASP played a crucial role in freeing male pilots for combat duty and contributing to the war effort.

After the war, the WASP were disbanded and their service largely forgotten by the public. They were not granted veteran status or benefits, and their contributions to the war effort went unrecognized for decades. Determined to rectify this injustice, Elaine Harmon and other former WASP began advocating for official recognition of their service and the awarding of veteran status.

For years, Harmon and her fellow WASP tirelessly lobbied Congress and the Department of Defense to acknowledge their service and grant them the recognition they deserved. Their efforts finally paid off in 1977 when President Jimmy Carter signed a law granting veteran status to the WASP.

However, it wasn't until many years later, in 2009, that the WASP were awarded the Congressional Gold Medal, the highest civilian honor bestowed by the United States Congress. The medal was presented to the WASP as a collective group in recognition of their pioneering service and contributions to the war effort.

Elaine Harmon's advocacy and determination played a crucial role in securing recognition for the WASP and ensuring that their legacy would be remembered and honored for generations to come. Her tireless efforts to fight for justice and equality for her fellow

WASP exemplified the spirit of service and sacrifice that defined their service during World War II.

74. Ulysses S. Grant

Ulysses S. Grant, born on April 27, 1822, in Point Pleasant, Ohio, was a prominent American military leader and the commanding general of the Union Army during the American Civil War. He played a pivotal role in leading the Union to victory in numerous battles, including the decisive Siege of Vicksburg.

Grant graduated from the United States Military Academy at West Point in 1843 and served with distinction in the Mexican-American War. After the war, he resigned from the military and pursued various civilian occupations, including farming and real estate, with limited success.

With the outbreak of the Civil War in 1861, Grant returned to military service and quickly rose through the ranks due to his strategic acumen and battlefield successes. In 1862, he won a series of important victories in the Western Theater, culminating in the capture of Forts Henry and Donelson and the Battle of Shiloh.

One of Grant's most significant achievements came in 1863 during the Siege of Vicksburg, a crucial Confederate stronghold on the Mississippi River. After a prolonged campaign, Grant's forces successfully besieged the city, cutting off its supply lines and forcing its surrender on July 4, 1863. The capture of Vicksburg was a turning point in the war, giving the Union control of the Mississippi River and splitting the Confederacy in two.

Grant's success at Vicksburg earned him national acclaim and led to his appointment as commanding general of the Union Army in March 1864. He devised a coordinated strategy to defeat the Confederacy, coordinating simultaneous offensives across multiple theaters of the war.

Under Grant's leadership, Union forces launched a series of successful campaigns, including the Overland Campaign in Virginia and the capture of Atlanta, Georgia. Despite heavy casualties, Grant's relentless pursuit of victory eventually wore down the Confederate forces and led to the surrender of General Robert E. Lee at Appomattox Court House on April 9, 1865, effectively ending the Civil War.

After the war, Grant served two terms as the 18th President of the United States from 1869 to 1877. He pursued policies aimed at promoting national reconciliation and Reconstruction in the South, although his administration faced challenges and controversies.

Ulysses S. Grant died on July 23, 1885.

75. Robert E. Lee

Robert E. Lee, born on January 19, 1807, in Stratford Hall, Virginia, was a prominent Confederate general known for his tactical brilliance and leadership during the American Civil War. He is best known for commanding the Confederate Army of Northern Virginia and leading it in major battles such as Gettysburg.

Lee graduated from the United States Military Academy at West Point in 1829 and served with distinction in the United States Army for over three decades. He gained valuable experience and earned a reputation as a skilled military engineer and officer during the Mexican-American War.

When the Civil War erupted in 1861, Lee faced a difficult decision: whether to remain loyal to the Union or join the Confederate cause. Despite his personal opposition to secession and slavery, Lee felt a strong allegiance to his home state of Virginia and chose to resign his commission in the U.S. Army to serve as a general in the Confederate Army.

Lee quickly rose to prominence as one of the Confederacy's most capable and respected military leaders. In June 1862, he assumed command of the Army of Northern Virginia, the principal Confederate army in the Eastern Theater of the war. Under Lee's leadership, the Army of Northern Virginia achieved several notable victories against the Union Army, including the Seven Days Battles, the Second Battle of Bull Run, and the Battle of Fredericksburg.

One of Lee's most famous and controversial campaigns occurred in the summer of 1863, when he led his army into Pennsylvania, culminating in the Battle of Gettysburg. The three-day battle resulted in a decisive Union victory and inflicted heavy casualties on both sides. Despite his tactical acumen, Lee's aggressive strategy ultimately failed to achieve its objectives, and the Confederate Army suffered significant losses.

Following the defeat at Gettysburg, Lee's army retreated back into Virginia, where they continued to engage in intense fighting against Union forces. Despite several more victories, including the Battle of Chancellorsville, Lee was unable to reverse the course of the war.

In April 1865, facing overwhelming odds and dwindling resources, Lee surrendered his army to Union General Ulysses S. Grant at Appomattox Court House, effectively ending the Civil War.

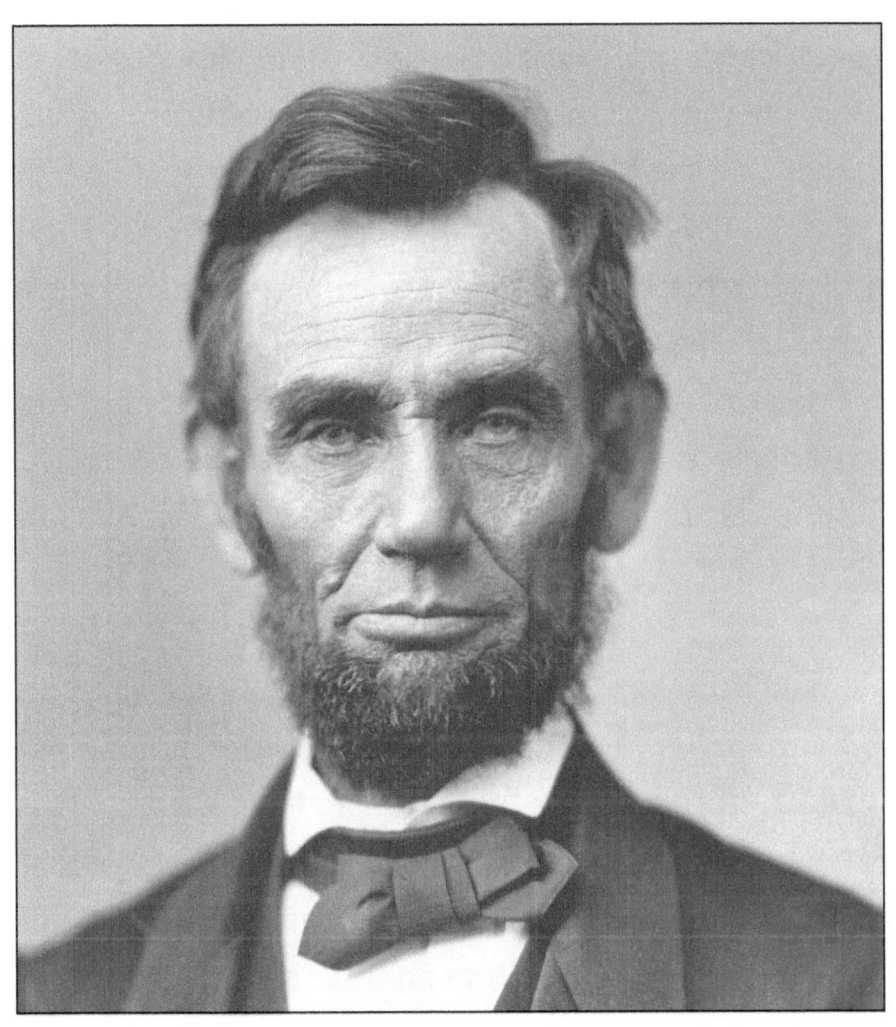

76. Abraham Lincoln

Abraham Lincoln, born on February 12, 1809, in a log cabin in Hardin County, Kentucky (now part of LaRue County), was the 16th President of the United States. He is best known for his leadership during the

American Civil War, his issuance of the Emancipation Proclamation, and his unwavering commitment to preserving the Union.

Lincoln's rise to the presidency came at a time of deep national division over the issue of slavery. With the election of Lincoln in 1860 as the first Republican president, many Southern states seceded from the Union, leading to the outbreak of the Civil War in April 1861.

Throughout his presidency, Lincoln's primary goal was to preserve the Union and restore peace to a nation torn apart by civil strife. Despite the tremendous challenges he faced, including intense political opposition and the staggering human cost of the war, Lincoln remained steadfast in his determination to achieve victory.

One of Lincoln's most significant actions during the war was the issuance of the Emancipation Proclamation on January 1, 1863. This executive order declared all enslaved people in Confederate-held territory to be free, transforming the Civil War into a struggle for freedom and emancipation.

While the Emancipation Proclamation did not immediately free all enslaved people, as it only applied to areas under Confederate control, it was a crucial step in advancing the cause of abolition and reshaping the moral and political landscape of the war. It also paved the way for the eventual passage of the 13th Amendment to the United States Constitution, which abolished slavery throughout the country.

In addition to his role as commander-in-chief and emancipator, Lincoln was also a skilled politician and statesman who navigated the complexities of wartime leadership with wisdom and foresight. He worked tirelessly to maintain support for the Union cause, rallying the American people with his eloquent speeches and steadfast resolve.

Tragically, Abraham Lincoln's life was cut short when he was assassinated by John Wilkes Booth, a Confederate sympathizer, on April 14, 1865, just days after the surrender of Confederate General Robert E. Lee at Appomattox Court House. Lincoln's death was a devastating blow to the nation, but his legacy as the "Great Emancipator" and the "Savior of the Union" endures.

Abraham Lincoln's leadership during one of the darkest periods in American history helped to preserve the Union, abolish slavery, and redefine the nation's commitment to liberty and equality for all its citizens.

77. William Tecumseh Sherman

William Tecumseh Sherman, born on February 8, 1820, in Lancaster, Ohio, was a prominent Union general during the American Civil War. He is best known for his innovative military strategies, including his "March to the Sea" campaign and the capture of Atlanta.

Sherman graduated from the United States Military Academy at West Point in 1840 and served in the United States Army for over a decade before resigning to pursue a career in banking and law. However, with the outbreak of the Civil War in 1861, Sherman returned to military service and quickly distinguished himself as a capable and aggressive commander.

One of Sherman's most significant contributions to the Union cause came in 1864 when he was appointed commander of the Military Division of the Mississippi, responsible for Union forces in the Western Theater of the war. Under Sherman's leadership, Union forces launched a series of successful campaigns aimed at defeating Confederate armies and securing control of key strategic objectives.

In the summer of 1864, Sherman embarked on his famous "March to the Sea," a bold and audacious campaign designed to cut a swath of destruction through the heart of the Confederacy and undermine its ability to wage war. Leading a force of over 60,000 troops, Sherman marched from Atlanta to Savannah, Georgia, leaving a path of destruction in his wake and depriving the Confederate army of vital resources.

The "March to the Sea" campaign was a devastating blow to the Confederacy and a turning point in the war. Sherman's forces inflicted heavy damage on

Confederate infrastructure, industry, and morale, hastening the collapse of the Confederate war effort.

In December 1864, Sherman's army captured Savannah, completing their march and effectively securing control of the Georgia coastline. The success of the campaign further bolstered Sherman's reputation as one of the Union's most effective and innovative commanders.

After the capture of Savannah, Sherman turned his sights northward and embarked on his famous "Carolinas Campaign," which aimed to disrupt Confederate supply lines and hasten the end of the war. In April 1865, Confederate General Joseph E. Johnston surrendered to Sherman near Durham, North Carolina, effectively ending the Civil War in the Eastern Theater.

78. Thomas Jonathan "Stonewall" Jackson

Thomas Jonathan "Stonewall" Jackson, born on January 21, 1824, in Clarksburg, Virginia (now West

Virginia), was a Confederate general known for his skilled tactics and leadership during the American Civil War. He earned his famous nickname "Stonewall" at the First Battle of Bull Run for his steadfast defense of his troops' position.

Jackson graduated from the United States Military Academy at West Point in 1846 and served in the United States Army during the Mexican-American War, where he earned a reputation for bravery and leadership. After the war, he resigned from the army to pursue a career in teaching at the Virginia Military Institute.

When the Civil War broke out in 1861, Jackson joined the Confederate cause and quickly rose through the ranks due to his military prowess and strategic brilliance. He earned his nickname "Stonewall" at the First Battle of Bull Run (First Manassas) in July 1861, where he and his troops stood firm against Union assaults, earning praise for their steadfastness in the face of adversity.

Jackson's military genius was further demonstrated in subsequent battles, where he employed bold and innovative tactics to achieve victory for the Confederacy. He became known for his aggressive and unpredictable maneuvers, often catching Union forces off guard and exploiting weaknesses in their defenses.

One of Jackson's most famous campaigns was the Shenandoah Valley Campaign of 1862, where he conducted a series of lightning-fast marches and surprise attacks against Union forces, earning him the admiration of his troops and the fear of his enemies. His success in the Shenandoah Valley helped to divert Union forces away from Richmond, the Confederate capital, and relieve pressure on Confederate forces in Virginia.

Jackson's most famous victory came at the Battle of Chancellorsville in May 1863, where he performed a daring flanking maneuver that routed a much larger Union army. However, his success was marred by tragedy when he was accidentally shot by his own men while scouting ahead of his lines. Jackson's left arm was amputated, and he died of complications from pneumonia eight days later on May 10, 1863.

79. Joshua Lawrence Chamberlain

Joshua Lawrence Chamberlain, born on September 8, 1828, in Brewer, Maine, was a Union Army officer known for his heroic defense of Little Round Top at the Battle of Gettysburg during the American Civil War. His actions played a crucial role in securing the Union left flank and ultimately contributed to the Union victory at Gettysburg.

Chamberlain was a respected academic and professor of rhetoric at Bowdoin College before the outbreak of the Civil War. In 1862, he left his teaching position to join the Union Army, enlisting as a lieutenant colonel in the 20th Maine Volunteer Infantry Regiment.

During the Battle of Gettysburg in July 1863, Chamberlain and his regiment were positioned on the extreme left flank of the Union line at Little Round Top, a strategic hill overlooking the battlefield. On the afternoon of July 2, Confederate forces launched a fierce assault on Little Round Top in an attempt to flank the Union position.

Chamberlain's regiment, positioned at the far end of the Union line, faced intense enemy pressure and was in danger of being overwhelmed. Recognizing the importance of holding their position, Chamberlain ordered a daring bayonet charge down the hill, leading his men in a desperate counterattack against the Confederate forces.

The charge was successful, driving back the Confederate attackers and securing the Union left flank. Chamberlain's decisive action at Little Round Top helped to stabilize the Union line and prevent a Confederate breakthrough, earning him widespread acclaim for his leadership and bravery.

For his heroism at Gettysburg, Chamberlain was promoted to brigadier general and later received the Medal of Honor, the highest military decoration awarded by the United States government. His defense of Little Round Top became one of the most celebrated episodes of the Civil War and cemented Chamberlain's reputation as one of the Union Army's most distinguished officers.

After the war, Chamberlain went on to serve as Governor of Maine and later as President of Bowdoin College. He remained active in veterans' affairs and Civil War commemorations, and his contributions to the Union cause were widely recognized and honored.

Joshua Lawrence Chamberlain died on February 24, 1914.

80. Clara Barton

Clara Barton, born on December 25, 1821, in North Oxford, Massachusetts, was a pioneering nurse, humanitarian, and founder of the American Red Cross. She is best known for her tireless efforts to provide medical care and assistance to wounded soldiers on the battlefield during the American Civil War.

Barton began her nursing career at a young age, caring for her brother David after he was seriously injured in a fall. She later worked as a teacher and clerk before finding her calling as a nurse during the Civil War.

In 1861, Barton volunteered as a nurse and began providing aid to wounded soldiers in Washington, D.C. She quickly gained a reputation for her compassion, dedication, and skill in tending to the sick and wounded.

Barton's most significant contributions came during some of the war's bloodiest battles, including the Battle of Antietam and the Battle of Fredericksburg, where she risked her life to provide medical care and comfort to soldiers on the front lines.

In addition to her work on the battlefield, Barton also organized relief efforts to provide supplies and assistance to soldiers and their families. She personally lobbied government officials and military leaders to improve medical care and sanitation conditions in military hospitals.

After the war, Barton continued her humanitarian work, focusing on helping locate missing soldiers and reuniting families separated by the conflict. She traveled to Europe, where she learned about the International Red Cross and its efforts to provide humanitarian aid during times of war and disaster.

Inspired by her experiences, Barton founded the American Red Cross in 1881, serving as its first president. Under her leadership, the organization grew rapidly, providing aid to victims of natural disasters, wars, and other emergencies both in the United States and around the world.

Clara Barton's legacy as a nurse, humanitarian, and founder of the American Red Cross continues to inspire people to this day. Her unwavering commitment to serving others, even in the face of great adversity, exemplifies the spirit of compassion and selflessness that defines the work of the Red Cross and other humanitarian organizations.

81. George Armstrong Custer

George Armstrong Custer, born on December 5, 1839, in New Rumley, Ohio, was a Union general known for his daring cavalry leadership during the American Civil War. He is best remembered for his role in several key battles, including his controversial actions at the Battle of Gettysburg.

Custer graduated from the United States Military Academy at West Point in 1861, just in time to join the Union Army at the outbreak of the Civil War. He quickly distinguished himself as a brave and aggressive officer, rising through the ranks to become one of the youngest generals in the Union Army.

During the Battle of Gettysburg in July 1863, Custer commanded the Michigan Cavalry Brigade, which played a crucial role in repelling Confederate cavalry attacks against the Union flanks. His decisive actions helped to secure victory for the Union forces and prevent a Confederate breakthrough.

Custer's most famous moment at Gettysburg came on the third day of the battle during Pickett's Charge, when he led a bold cavalry charge against Confederate infantry positions on the Union right flank. Although the charge was ultimately unsuccessful and resulted in heavy casualties, Custer's bravery and leadership earned him widespread acclaim and admiration.

After Gettysburg, Custer continued to serve with distinction in the Union Army, participating in several major campaigns and battles, including the Overland Campaign and the Siege of Petersburg. He also played a prominent role in the Appomattox Campaign, which led to the surrender of Confederate General Robert E. Lee and the end of the Civil War.

Following the war, Custer remained in the military and continued to serve on the western frontier. He is perhaps best known for his involvement in the Indian Wars, particularly his defeat at the Battle of the Little Bighorn in 1876, where he and his entire command were killed by Lakota Sioux and Cheyenne warriors.

82. Jefferson Davis

Jefferson Davis, born on June 3, 1808, in Fairview, Kentucky, was a prominent American politician and the President of the Confederate States of America during the American Civil War. He played a central role in the formation and leadership of the Confederacy, guiding the Southern states through the tumultuous years of the Civil War.

Davis graduated from the United States Military Academy at West Point in 1828 and served as an officer in the United States Army before embarking on a career in politics. He served as a U.S. Senator and Secretary of War under President Franklin Pierce before resigning to become the President of the Confederate States of America.

In February 1861, following the secession of several Southern states in response to Abraham Lincoln's election as President of the United States, Davis was chosen as the provisional president of the Confederate States. He was later elected to a six-year term as the permanent president in November 1861.

As president of the Confederacy, Davis faced numerous challenges, including organizing a new government, managing the Confederate economy and military, and rallying public support for the Southern cause. He struggled to maintain unity among the Confederate states and faced criticism for his handling of military strategy and government affairs.

Davis's leadership during the Civil War was marked by both successes and failures. While he was praised for his dedication to the Confederate cause and his efforts to mobilize Southern resources for the war effort, he also faced criticism for his management of the Confederate military and his handling of internal political disputes.

Ultimately, the Confederacy was defeated in the Civil War, and Davis was captured by Union forces in May 1865. He was imprisoned for two years before being released on bail and later pardoned by President Andrew Johnson.

After the war, Davis retired to private life and spent his remaining years writing and speaking on behalf of the Southern cause. He died on December 6, 1889, in New Orleans, Louisiana.

83. Winfield Scott Hancock

Winfield Scott Hancock, born on February 14, 1824, in Montgomery Square, Pennsylvania, was a prominent Union general known for his leadership during the American Civil War. He played a significant role in several key battles, including his command at the Battle of Gettysburg, where he distinguished himself during Pickett's Charge.

Hancock graduated from the United States Military Academy at West Point in 1844 and served in the United States Army before the outbreak of the Civil War. He quickly rose through the ranks, earning a reputation as a skilled and courageous officer.

At the Battle of Gettysburg in July 1863, Hancock served as the commander of the Union II Corps, a position that placed him at the center of the Union defensive line on Cemetery Ridge. On the third day of the battle, Confederate General Robert E. Lee launched a massive infantry assault known as Pickett's Charge against the center of the Union line.

Recognizing the critical importance of holding their position, Hancock personally directed the Union defenses and inspired his troops to stand firm in the face of the Confederate onslaught. Despite being wounded during the battle, Hancock remained on the front lines, rallying his men and coordinating their defense.

Hancock's leadership and courage during Pickett's Charge helped to repulse the Confederate attack and secure victory for the Union forces at Gettysburg. His decisive actions on the battlefield earned him widespread praise and admiration from his fellow officers and troops.

After Gettysburg, Hancock continued to serve with distinction in the Union Army, participating in several other major campaigns and battles, including the Overland Campaign and the Siege of Petersburg. He also played a prominent role in the Appomattox Campaign, which led to the surrender of Confederate General Robert E. Lee and the end of the Civil War.

Following the war, Hancock pursued a career in politics and briefly served as the Democratic nominee for President of the United States in 1880. However, he was narrowly defeated by Republican candidate James A. Garfield.

Winfield Scott Hancock died on February 9, 1886.

84. Michael Jordan

Michael Jordan, born on February 17, 1963, in Brooklyn, New York, is a former professional basketball player widely regarded as one of the greatest athletes of all time. Known for his exceptional talent, competitive spirit, and unparalleled success on the basketball court, Jordan achieved legendary status during his career with the Chicago Bulls in the NBA.

Jordan's basketball journey began at a young age, and he quickly emerged as a standout player in high school and college. He gained national attention during his tenure at the University of North Carolina, where he helped lead the Tar Heels to a national championship in 1982.

In 1984, Jordan entered the NBA draft and was selected by the Chicago Bulls as the third overall pick. From the moment he stepped onto the court as a professional, Jordan made an immediate impact, showcasing his extraordinary athleticism, scoring ability, and defensive prowess.

Throughout his illustrious career, Jordan dominated the NBA like few others before him. He won six NBA championships with the Chicago Bulls, earning NBA Finals MVP honors each time. His relentless work ethic, determination, and clutch performances in crucial moments earned him the nickname "His Airness" and made him a cultural icon around the world.

Jordan's list of accolades is extensive and includes five regular-season MVP awards, 14 NBA All-Star selections, and 10 scoring titles, among numerous other honors. He also played a pivotal role in popularizing the game of basketball globally, helping to elevate the NBA to unprecedented levels of popularity and paving the way for future generations of basketball players.

Beyond his on-court achievements, Jordan's impact extends far beyond basketball. He became a global brand ambassador and one of the most recognizable faces in sports, with his iconic Air Jordan sneakers and endorsements making him one of the wealthiest athletes in history.

After retiring from basketball for the second time in 2003, Jordan transitioned into a successful career as a businessman and owner of the Charlotte Hornets NBA franchise. Despite his retirement from playing, Jordan's influence on the game of basketball and his status as a cultural icon continue to resonate with fans worldwide, cementing his legacy as one of the greatest athletes of all time.

85. Muhammad Ali

Muhammad Ali, born Cassius Marcellus Clay Jr., is widely regarded as one of the greatest athletes of all time, known for his exceptional boxing skills, remarkable athleticism, and unparalleled achievements in the ring. Throughout his illustrious career, Ali accomplished feats that solidified his legacy as a boxing icon and earned him a place among the most celebrated athletes in history.

Ali burst onto the professional boxing scene in the early 1960s with a meteoric rise fueled by his remarkable talent and charismatic personality. He won the Olympic gold medal in the light heavyweight division at the 1960 Rome Olympics, foreshadowing the greatness he would achieve in the years to come.

In 1964, Ali stunned the world by defeating Sonny Liston to capture the world heavyweight championship at just 22 years old. It was the beginning of an extraordinary journey that would see him become the first fighter to win the heavyweight title three times.

Ali's boxing style was characterized by his lightning-fast footwork, razor-sharp jab, and unparalleled defensive skills. He possessed a rare combination of speed, agility, and power that allowed him to dominate opponents both inside and outside the ring.

One of Ali's most famous fights came in 1971 when he faced Joe Frazier in the "Fight of the Century." The bout, billed as a showdown between two undefeated heavyweight champions, captivated the world and lived up to its hype as a brutal and epic battle. Despite suffering his first professional defeat, Ali's resilience and determination in the ring solidified his reputation as a boxing legend.

In 1974, Ali reclaimed the world heavyweight championship by defeating George Foreman in the historic "Rumble in the Jungle" in Kinshasa, Zaire. In a stunning display of strategy and skill, Ali employed his now-legendary "rope-a-dope" tactic to tire out Foreman before knocking him out in the eighth round, reclaiming the title and proving his greatness once again.

Ali's illustrious career culminated in his thrilling trilogy of fights with Joe Frazier and his epic battles with other boxing legends such as Ken Norton and Larry Holmes. He retired from boxing in 1981 with a professional record of 56 wins and only 5 losses, cementing his status as one of the greatest boxers of all time.

86. Jackie Robinson

Jackie Robinson, born on January 31, 1919, in Cairo, Georgia, was a trailblazing baseball player who made history by breaking the color barrier in Major League Baseball (MLB). His courageous actions and remarkable talent paved the way for integration in professional sports and inspired generations of athletes.

Robinson's journey to the major leagues was marked by adversity and perseverance. Despite facing racial discrimination and barriers throughout his career, he excelled as a multi-sport athlete at UCLA, where he became the first student-athlete to letter in four sports: baseball, basketball, football, and track.

In 1945, Robinson signed a contract with the Kansas City Monarchs of the Negro Leagues, where he showcased his exceptional talent as a versatile player. His performance caught the attention of Branch Rickey, the general manager of the Brooklyn Dodgers, who saw in Robinson the potential to challenge baseball's segregation policies.

On April 15, 1947, Jackie Robinson made history when he stepped onto the field as the starting first baseman for the Brooklyn Dodgers, becoming the first African American to play in the major leagues in the modern era. Robinson's integration of MLB was a groundbreaking moment in American sports and a significant milestone in the civil rights movement.

Despite facing intense racial hostility from fans, opposing players, and even some teammates, Robinson remained steadfast in his commitment to excellence and dignity. His exceptional skills as a hitter, fielder, and baserunner helped him earn the respect of his peers and fans alike, and he quickly established himself as one of the game's premier players.

In his rookie season, Robinson won the inaugural Rookie of the Year Award and played a key role in leading the Dodgers to the National League pennant. He went on to have a distinguished career, earning six All-Star selections, winning the National League MVP award in 1949, and helping the Dodgers win their first World Series championship in 1955.

Jackie Robinson retired from baseball in 1956, but his impact on the game and society endured long after his playing days ended. In 1962, he was inducted into the Baseball Hall of Fame.

87. Babe Ruth

Babe Ruth, born George Herman Ruth Jr. on February 6, 1895, in Baltimore, Maryland, is widely regarded as one of the greatest baseball players of all time. Known for his legendary home run hitting, charismatic personality, and larger-than-life persona, Ruth became an American icon and transformed the game of baseball during his illustrious career.

Ruth began his professional baseball career as a pitcher for the Boston Red Sox in 1914, where he quickly gained attention for his exceptional pitching ability. However, it was his prowess as a hitter that would ultimately define his legacy and revolutionize the sport.

In 1919, Ruth was traded to the New York Yankees, where he transitioned from a dominant pitcher to a full-time outfielder and became the most feared hitter in baseball. Ruth's unprecedented power and ability to hit towering home runs captured the imagination of fans and earned him the nickname "The Sultan of Swat."

Throughout the 1920s, Ruth's prodigious home run hitting captivated the nation and helped transform baseball into America's pastime. He shattered numerous records and established himself as the game's premier slugger, setting single-season home run records and leading the league in home runs year after year.

One of Ruth's most iconic achievements came in 1927 when he hit 60 home runs in a single season, a record that stood for nearly four decades. His prodigious power and offensive prowess helped lead the Yankees to multiple World Series championships, solidifying his status as a baseball legend.

Beyond his on-field exploits, Ruth's larger-than-life personality and off-field antics made him a cultural phenomenon. He was known for his flamboyant lifestyle, colorful quotes, and love of the spotlight, making him one of the most recognizable and beloved figures of his era.

Despite his larger-than-life persona, Ruth was also a remarkably skilled and disciplined athlete. He possessed a keen understanding of the game and was known for his strategic approach to hitting, as well as his ability to perform under pressure in clutch situations.

He retired from baseball in 1935. Babe Ruth was elected to the Baseball Hall of Fame in 1936 as one of its inaugural inductees.

88. Jim Thorpe

Jim Thorpe, born on May 28, 1888, near Prague, Oklahoma, was a legendary multi-sport athlete who achieved unparalleled success in several sports, including track and field, football, and baseball. His remarkable athletic ability, versatility, and competitive spirit made him one of the most celebrated athletes of the 20th century.

Thorpe's journey to athletic greatness began during his childhood on the Sac and Fox Indian Reservation in Oklahoma, where he honed his athletic skills playing traditional Native American games. He attended the Carlisle Indian Industrial School in

Pennsylvania, where he excelled as a multi-sport athlete under the guidance of renowned coach Glenn "Pop" Warner.

In 1912, Thorpe represented the United States at the Olympic Games in Stockholm, Sweden, where he achieved legendary status by winning gold medals in both the pentathlon and decathlon. His dominant performances in track and field earned him widespread acclaim and established him as one of the greatest athletes of his time.

Following his Olympic success, Thorpe turned his attention to professional sports, where he continued to excel as a multi-sport athlete. He played professional football for several teams, including the Canton Bulldogs, where he helped lead the team to multiple championships and solidified his reputation as one of the greatest football players of his era.

In addition to football, Thorpe also had a successful career in professional baseball, playing for teams in the Major Leagues and minor leagues. His versatility and athleticism made him a standout player on the baseball diamond, and he became known for his powerful hitting and exceptional fielding abilities.

Throughout his athletic career, Thorpe faced numerous challenges and obstacles, including discrimination and prejudice due to his Native American heritage. Despite these challenges, he persevered and achieved remarkable success, leaving an indelible mark on the world of sports.

In recognition of his extraordinary athletic achievements, Jim Thorpe was named the greatest athlete of the first half of the 20th century by the Associated Press in 1950.

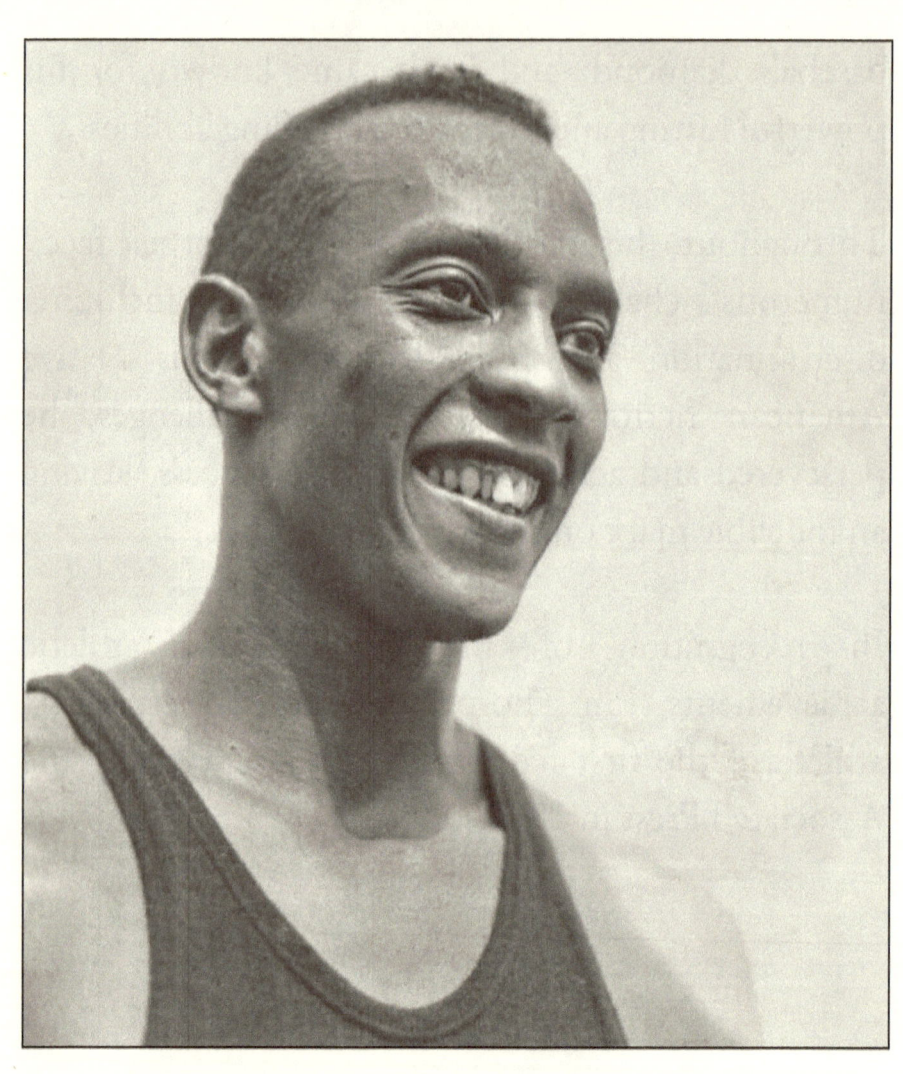

89. Jesse Owens

Jesse Owens, born James Cleveland Owens on September 12, 1913, in Oakville, Alabama, was a legendary track and field athlete whose remarkable achievements transcended sports and had profound cultural significance. Best known for his historic performance at the 1936 Olympic Games in Berlin, Owens defied racial prejudice and shattered Adolf Hitler's notions of Aryan supremacy by winning four gold medals in track and field events.

Owens' journey to Olympic glory began during his college years at Ohio State University, where he quickly emerged as one of the most talented athletes in the nation. In 1935, he set three world records and tied another in less than an hour at the Big Ten track and field championships, a feat that remains unparalleled in the history of the sport.

The pinnacle of Owens' athletic career came at the 1936 Olympic Games in Berlin, Germany, where he delivered a series of electrifying performances that captivated the world. Despite facing intense racial discrimination and pressure, Owens won gold medals in the 100 meters, 200 meters, long jump, and 4x100 meters relay, becoming the first American track and field athlete to win four gold medals in a single Olympic Games.

Owens' triumph in Berlin was not only a personal victory but also a powerful rebuke to Hitler's ideology of Aryan supremacy and racial superiority. His dominant performance on the world stage shattered racial stereotypes and inspired people around the globe, reaffirming the power of sports to transcend social and political barriers.

Despite his extraordinary achievements, Owens returned to a segregated America where he continued to face racial discrimination and inequality. However, he remained a symbol of hope and resilience, using his platform to advocate for civil rights and equality for all.

In the decades following his Olympic triumph, Owens' legacy continued to resonate, earning him numerous accolades and honors, including induction into the U.S. Olympic Hall of Fame and the Track and Field Hall of Fame. His remarkable achievements and enduring impact on sports and society have cemented his status as one of the most iconic and influential athletes in history.

90. Tom Brady

Tom Brady, born on August 3, 1977, in San Mateo, California, is an American football quarterback widely regarded as one of the greatest players in the history of the National Football League (NFL). Known for his exceptional talent, leadership, and unparalleled success on the gridiron, Brady has achieved legendary status throughout his illustrious career.

Brady's journey to NFL stardom began at the University of Michigan, where he played college football for the Wolverines before being selected by the New England Patriots in the sixth round of the 2000 NFL Draft. Despite being a relatively unheralded prospect, Brady quickly established himself as a key player for the Patriots and soon emerged as one of the league's premier quarterbacks.

Over the course of his career, Brady has amassed an impressive list of accomplishments, including multiple Super Bowl victories, MVP awards, and Pro Bowl selections. His unparalleled success on the field has earned him widespread acclaim and recognition as one of the most dominant players in NFL history.

One of Brady's defining characteristics as a quarterback is his unparalleled competitiveness and clutch performances in high-pressure situations. He has a knack for delivering in critical moments, earning him the nickname "The Comeback Kid" for his ability to engineer late-game rallies and dramatic victories.

Brady's legacy as one of the greatest quarterbacks of all time was further solidified during his tenure with the New England Patriots, where he won six Super Bowl championships, the most by any player in NFL history. His partnership with Patriots head coach Bill Belichick formed one of the most successful dynasties in NFL history, with the duo leading the team to numerous division titles, conference championships, and Super Bowl appearances.

In 2020, Brady signed with the Tampa Bay Buccaneers, where he continued to defy expectations and add to his legacy. In his first season with the Buccaneers, Brady led the team to victory in Super Bowl LV, earning his seventh Super Bowl ring and further cementing his status as one of the greatest quarterbacks of all time.

Beyond his on-field achievements, Brady is also known for his leadership, work ethic, and dedication to his craft. He is revered by teammates, coaches, and fans alike for his relentless pursuit of excellence and commitment to winning.

91. Michael Johnson

Michael Johnson, born on September 13, 1967, in Dallas, Texas, is a legendary track and field athlete who is widely regarded as one of the greatest sprinters in the history of the sport. Known for his distinctive upright running style, Johnson achieved unparalleled success in the 200-meter and 400-meter sprints, setting multiple world records and winning numerous Olympic and World Championship titles.

Johnson's dominance on the track began during his collegiate career at Baylor University, where he won multiple NCAA titles and earned a reputation as one of the most talented sprinters in the nation. In 1991, he burst onto the international scene by winning the 200 meters at the World Championships in Tokyo, Japan, establishing himself as a force to be reckoned with on the world stage.

One of Johnson's most iconic achievements came at the 1996 Olympic Games in Atlanta, Georgia, where he made history by becoming the first man to win gold medals in both the 200 meters and 400 meters at the same Olympics. His electrifying performances in Atlanta captivated the world and solidified his status as one of the greatest sprinters of all time.

In addition to his Olympic success, Johnson also set multiple world records in the 200 meters and 400 meters during his career. In 1996, he set the world record in the 200 meters with a time of 19.32 seconds, a mark that stood for over a decade before being broken. He also set the world record in the 400 meters with a time of 43.18 seconds in 1999, a record that remains unbroken to this day.

Johnson's unparalleled speed, power, and technical prowess revolutionized the sport of track and field and inspired generations of athletes around the world.

His distinctive running style, characterized by his upright posture and powerful strides, became his trademark and set him apart from his competitors.

Throughout his career, Johnson remained a dominant force in sprinting, earning numerous accolades and honors, including multiple Olympic gold medals, World Championship titles, and Athlete of the Year awards. He retired from competitive athletics in 2001.

92. Dan Gable

Dan Gable, born on October 25, 1948, in Waterloo, Iowa, is a legendary wrestler and coach who is widely regarded as one of the greatest competitors in the history of collegiate and Olympic wrestling. Known for his unparalleled work ethic, technical expertise, and relentless determination, Gable achieved unparalleled success both as an athlete and as a coach, leaving an indelible mark on the sport of wrestling.

Gable's wrestling career began during his high school years at Waterloo West High School, where he quickly emerged as one of the most talented and dominant wrestlers in the state of Iowa. He compiled an astonishing record of 64-0 and won two state championships, establishing himself as a force to be reckoned with on the mat.

After high school, Gable continued his wrestling career at Iowa State University, where he achieved unprecedented success as a collegiate wrestler. He compiled an astonishing record of 181-1 and won two NCAA championships, earning a reputation as one of the most dominant wrestlers in NCAA history.

However, Gable's most iconic achievement came at the 1972 Olympic Games in Munich, Germany, where he won a gold medal in freestyle wrestling in the 68 kg weight class. His dominant performance in Munich solidified his status as one of the greatest wrestlers of his generation and earned him widespread acclaim and recognition.

Following his Olympic triumph, Gable transitioned to coaching, where he continued to make an indelible impact on the sport of wrestling. He served as the head wrestling coach at the University of Iowa for over two decades, leading the Hawkeyes to unprecedented success and establishing them as a powerhouse program in collegiate wrestling.

Under Gable's guidance, the University of Iowa won 15 NCAA team championships and produced numerous individual national champions and Olympic medalists. His relentless focus on discipline, hard work, and mental toughness have helped mold generations of wrestlers.

93. Jerry Rice

Jerry Rice, born on October 13, 1962, in Starkville, Mississippi, is a legendary American football wide receiver who is widely regarded as one of the greatest players in the history of the National Football League (NFL). Known for his exceptional talent, work ethic, and longevity, Rice achieved unparalleled success on the gridiron and left an indelible mark on the sport of football.

Rice's journey to NFL stardom began at Mississippi Valley State University, where he emerged as one of the most dominant wide receivers in college football history. Despite playing at a small school, Rice's extraordinary talent and production caught the attention of NFL scouts, and he was selected by the San Francisco 49ers in the first round of the 1985 NFL Draft.

Over the course of his illustrious NFL career, Rice established himself as the premier wide receiver of his era and set numerous records that still stand to this day. He was known for his precise route-running, exceptional hands, and unparalleled work ethic, which allowed him to thrive in an era known for physical play and defensive dominance.

Rice's list of accolades and accomplishments is extensive and includes three Super Bowl championships, 13 Pro Bowl selections, and numerous All-Pro honors. He also holds numerous NFL records, including most career receptions, receiving yards, and touchdown receptions, making him one of the most statistically dominant players in league history.

One of Rice's most memorable performances came in Super Bowl XXIII in 1989, where he earned MVP honors after catching 11 passes for 215 yards and a touchdown to lead the 49ers to victory over the Cincinnati Bengals. His clutch play and ability to perform on the biggest stage solidified his reputation as one of the greatest players in NFL history.

Beyond his on-field achievements, Rice was also known for his unparalleled work ethic and dedication to his craft. He was renowned for his rigorous training regimen and tireless commitment to improving his game, setting a standard of excellence that continues to inspire athletes across all sports.

In addition to his success with the 49ers, Rice also had productive stints with the Oakland Raiders and the Seattle Seahawks before retiring from the NFL in 2005. He was inducted into the Pro Football Hall of Fame in 2010.

94. Florence Griffith Joyner

Florence Griffith Joyner, born on December 21, 1959, in Los Angeles, California, was a trailblazing track and field athlete known for her electrifying speed, exceptional athleticism, and iconic style. Widely regarded as one of the greatest sprinters in the history of the sport, Griffith Joyner achieved unprecedented success on the track and left an indelible mark on the world of athletics.

Griffith Joyner's journey to track and field stardom began during her collegiate years at California State University, Northridge, where she competed as a member of the track and field team. She quickly emerged as a standout performer, earning All-American honors and capturing multiple conference championships in the sprints and the long jump.

However, it was during the 1988 Olympic Games in Seoul, South Korea, that Griffith Joyner achieved her greatest success and etched her name into the annals of track and field history. At the age of 28, she delivered a series of electrifying performances that captivated the world and solidified her status as one of the most dominant athletes of her generation.

Griffith Joyner's most iconic moment came in the 1988 Olympic final of the women's 100 meters, where she shattered the world record with a stunning time of

10.49 seconds, a mark that still stands as the fastest time ever recorded by a woman. She followed up this remarkable performance with another gold medal in the 200 meters, setting a world record of 21.34 seconds that remains unbroken to this day.

In addition to her extraordinary speed, Griffith Joyner was also known for her flamboyant and colorful racing outfits, which featured vibrant colors, bold patterns, and one-legged bodysuits. Her unique sense of style and fashion sense made her a cultural icon and helped elevate the profile of women's track and field on the global stage.

Florence Griffith Joyner died in her sleep, aged 36, in 1998.

95. Hank Aaron

Hank Aaron, born on February 5, 1934, in Mobile, Alabama, was a legendary baseball player known for his remarkable talent, unwavering perseverance, and enduring legacy in the sport. Widely regarded as one of the greatest players in the history of Major League

Baseball (MLB), Aaron's illustrious career spanned over two decades and left an indelible mark on the game.

Aaron's journey to baseball stardom began in the Negro Leagues, where he played for the Indianapolis Clowns before being signed by the Milwaukee Braves in 1952. He made his MLB debut with the Braves in 1954 and quickly established himself as one of the premier hitters in the league, earning his first of 25 All-Star selections in his rookie season.

Throughout his career, Aaron was known for his exceptional hitting ability, power, and consistency at the plate. He finished his career with 3,771 hits, 755 home runs, and 2,297 runs batted in, cementing his place among the all-time leaders in those categories. His 755 home runs stood as the MLB record for over three decades until it was surpassed by Barry Bonds in 2007.

One of Aaron's most iconic achievements came on April 8, 1974, when he broke Babe Ruth's long-standing record of 714 career home runs. Aaron's milestone home run, hit off Los Angeles Dodgers pitcher Al Downing, remains one of the most celebrated moments in baseball history and solidified his status as a living legend.

Despite facing racism and discrimination throughout his career, Aaron remained steadfast in his pursuit of excellence and became a symbol of resilience and perseverance for generations of athletes. His dignified demeanor, quiet determination, and unwavering commitment to his craft earned him widespread respect and admiration both on and off the field.

After retiring as a player, Aaron remained active in baseball as a front-office executive and ambassador for the sport. He was inducted into the Baseball Hall of Fame in 1982, further solidifying his legacy as one of the greatest players to ever step foot on the diamond.

96. Wilma Rudolph

Wilma Rudolph, born on June 23, 1940, in Saint Bethlehem, Tennessee, overcame numerous obstacles to become one of the most celebrated athletes in the history of track and field. Afflicted with polio as a child, Rudolph defied the odds and went on to achieve remarkable success on the track, culminating in her historic performance at the 1960 Olympic Games in Rome.

Rudolph's journey to Olympic glory began in her hometown of Clarksville, Tennessee, where she first discovered her passion for running. Despite facing physical challenges due to her bout with polio, Rudolph was determined to excel in athletics and began training under the guidance of her high school track coach, Ed Temple.

At the 1960 Olympic Games in Rome, Rudolph's talent and perseverance were on full display as she captured the hearts of millions around the world with her electrifying performances on the track. She made history by becoming the first American woman to win three gold medals in a single Olympic Games, dominating the sprint events with victories in the 100 meters, 200 meters, and 4x100 meters relay.

Rudolph's Olympic triumphs not only solidified her status as one of the greatest sprinters of her generation but also inspired countless individuals around the world with her remarkable journey of resilience and determination. She became a symbol of hope and perseverance, breaking down barriers and paving the way for future generations of female athletes.

In addition to her Olympic success, Rudolph continued to make an impact on the track and field world, setting numerous world records and earning countless accolades throughout her career. She retired from competitive athletics in 1962 but remained actively involved in the sport as a coach, mentor, and advocate for women's rights and equality in sports.

97. Jimmie Johnson

Jimmie Johnson, born on September 17, 1975, in El Cajon, California, is a legendary NASCAR driver who has left an indelible mark on the world of auto racing. Throughout his illustrious career, Johnson has achieved unprecedented success on the track, earning widespread acclaim and cementing his legacy as one of the greatest drivers in NASCAR history.

Johnson's journey to NASCAR stardom began in the early 2000s when he joined Hendrick Motorsports, one of the premier teams in the sport. He quickly established himself as a formidable competitor, earning his first NASCAR Cup Series victory in 2002 at the Auto Club Speedway.

However, it was in the mid-2000s that Johnson's career truly took off, as he embarked on a historic run of dominance that would solidify his status as a NASCAR legend. From 2006 to 2010, Johnson captured an unprecedented five consecutive NASCAR Cup Series championships, a feat that had never been accomplished before in the sport's storied history.

One of the highlights of Johnson's career came in 2006 when he won his first Daytona 500, NASCAR's most prestigious race. Held annually at the Daytona International Speedway in Florida, the Daytona 500 is known for its high speeds, intense competition, and thrilling finishes. Johnson's victory in the "Great American Race" further cemented his status as a superstar in the world of auto racing.

Throughout his career, Johnson has amassed an impressive list of accomplishments, including 83 NASCAR Cup Series victories, making him one of the winningest drivers in the history of the sport. He has also earned numerous accolades and awards, including seven NASCAR Cup Series championships, tying him with legends Richard Petty and Dale Earnhardt for the most titles in NASCAR history.

In addition to his success on the track, Johnson is also known for his philanthropic efforts and contributions to the community.

98. Mark Spitz

Mark Spitz, born on February 10, 1950, in Modesto, California, is a legendary swimmer who achieved unparalleled success in the sport of swimming during the 1972 Olympic Games in Munich, Germany. Spitz's dominance in the pool and his remarkable performances at the Olympics solidified his legacy as one of the greatest swimmers in history.

At the age of 18, Spitz burst onto the international swimming scene at the 1968 Olympic Games in Mexico City, where he won two gold medals, a silver, and a bronze. Despite his impressive debut, it was at the 1972 Olympics in Munich that Spitz would etch his name into the annals of Olympic history.

During the 1972 Games, Spitz delivered a breathtaking display of speed and skill, capturing the imagination of fans around the world with his remarkable performances in the pool. Over the course of the Olympics, Spitz won an unprecedented seven gold medals, setting world records in all seven events in which he competed.

Spitz's seven gold medals at the 1972 Olympics stood as a record for decades and solidified his status as one of the greatest Olympians of all time. His achievements in Munich propelled him to international superstardom and made him a household name around the world.

In addition to his success at the Olympics, Spitz also enjoyed a highly successful swimming career outside of the Games. He set numerous world records and won multiple national and international championships, establishing himself as one of the most dominant swimmers of his era.

After retiring from competitive swimming, Spitz remained active in the sport as a coach, commentator, and ambassador. He continued to inspire future generations of swimmers with his remarkable achievements and dedication to excellence in the pool.

99. Balto and the Serum Run to Nome

In the winter of 1925, the remote town of Nome, Alaska, faced a dire medical emergency. An outbreak of diphtheria, a highly contagious bacterial infection, threatened the lives of its inhabitants, particularly the children. With no antitoxin serum available in Nome, the situation grew increasingly desperate as the disease spread rapidly.

In a race against time, a daring plan was devised to transport the life-saving serum from Anchorage to Nome, a distance of nearly 700 miles, using a relay of dog sled teams. The treacherous journey would traverse harsh and unforgiving terrain, including frozen tundra, steep mountain passes, and treacherous sea ice.

Leading one of the sled teams was Balto, a Siberian Husky with a reputation for strength, endurance, and intelligence. Alongside his musher, Norwegian-born Leonhard Seppala, and a team of brave sled dogs, Balto embarked on the final leg of the perilous journey.

Despite facing blizzard conditions and sub-zero temperatures, Balto and his team pressed on, navigating through the darkness and howling winds. Guided by Seppala's expert handling and Balto's keen instincts, they raced against time to deliver the precious cargo to Nome.

Finally, on February 2, 1925, after an arduous journey of more than 20 hours, Balto and his team arrived in Nome, greeted by a relieved and grateful community. Their heroic efforts had successfully delivered the life-saving serum, helping to halt the spread of the deadly disease and saving countless lives.

Balto's courage and determination captured the hearts of people around the world, earning him widespread acclaim and recognition. He became an overnight sensation, hailed as a symbol of hope and resilience in the face of adversity.

His legacy lives on through statues, memorials, and the annual Iditarod Trail Sled Dog Race, which commemorates the historic Serum Run to Nome.

Today, Balto's story serves as a reminder of the remarkable bond between humans and animals, as well as the extraordinary feats that can be achieved through teamwork, perseverance, and courage in the face of adversity. Balto remains a true American hero.

100. Cher Ami, the Pigeon Messenger

In the tumultuous trenches of World War I, amidst the chaos and carnage of battle, one unlikely hero emerged to deliver a message of hope and salvation to beleaguered soldiers. Cher Ami, a carrier pigeon serving with the U.S. Army Signal Corps, would become a symbol of bravery and resilience in the face of adversity.

The year was 1918, and the "Lost Battalion," a unit of American soldiers isolated deep behind enemy lines in the Argonne Forest of France, found themselves surrounded by German forces. Cut off from friendly lines and running low on supplies, the situation grew increasingly dire as the enemy closed in.

Desperate for reinforcements and supplies, the commanding officer of the Lost Battalion turned to Cher Ami, a trusted carrier pigeon trained to deliver messages under fire. Secured in a small canister attached to his leg, Cher Ami carried the crucial message pleading for assistance and signaling the battalion's exact location.

As Cher Ami took flight amidst a hail of enemy gunfire, tragedy struck. Shot through the breast and blinded in one eye, the courageous pigeon refused to falter, pressing on with unwavering determination. Dodging bullets and fighting through pain, Cher Ami soared above the battlefield, his mission clear and his resolve unshaken.

Miraculously, Cher Ami reached his destination, delivering the life-saving message to Allied forces and guiding them to the trapped soldiers of the Lost Battalion. His courageous actions allowed for the successful rescue of nearly 200 soldiers, who otherwise faced certain death or capture by the enemy.

Cher Ami's bravery and sacrifice captured the hearts and imaginations of people around the world. His daring flight under fire became a symbol of hope and resilience, inspiring both soldiers on the front lines and civilians on the home front.

For his extraordinary service, Cher Ami was awarded the French Croix de Guerre for bravery, becoming one of the few non-human recipients of the prestigious military honor. He was a glowing example of courage, loyalty, and sacrifice, reminding us that heroes come in all shapes and sizes, even those with feathers and wings.

101. Smoky the War Dog

In the midst of the chaos and uncertainty of World War II, an unlikely hero emerged, bringing comfort, companionship, and courage to soldiers on the front lines. Smoky, a Yorkshire Terrier with a heart as big as her diminutive stature, would become a beloved mascot and invaluable asset to the U.S. Army during the Pacific Theater campaign.

Smoky's journey began when she was found by American soldier Corporal William Wynne in the jungles of New Guinea. Instantly bonding with the tiny dog, Wynne adopted her as his own and soon discovered her remarkable intelligence, loyalty, and fearlessness.

As Wynne's faithful companion, Smoky quickly endeared herself to the soldiers of the 5th Air Force, providing much-needed morale boosts and moments of joy amidst the hardships of war. Her cheerful demeanor and affectionate nature brought solace to weary soldiers and lifted their spirits during the darkest of times.

But Smoky's contributions to the war effort went beyond mere companionship. Her small size and agility made her uniquely suited for tasks that larger animals could not accomplish. In particular, Smoky's ability to crawl through narrow underground pipes proved invaluable for laying communication lines and detecting hidden enemy positions.

During one harrowing mission, Smoky's keen senses detected an enemy attack and alerted soldiers to the impending danger, saving countless lives in the process. Her bravery and quick thinking under fire earned her the admiration and gratitude of her fellow soldiers, who affectionately dubbed her the "War Dog."

Throughout the war, Smoky remained by Wynne's side, accompanying him on numerous combat missions and enduring the hardships of jungle warfare without complaint. Her unwavering loyalty and steadfast courage served as an inspiration to all who knew her, proving that even the smallest among us can make a profound impact on history.

After the war, Smoky continued to bring joy and comfort to those around her, becoming a beloved therapy dog and celebrity in her own right. Her remarkable story shows us the enduring bond between humans and animals and the power of courage and companionship in times of adversity.

The End

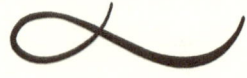

Other Books from Seniorality

To find your next book visit:
www.amazon.com/author/seniorality
Where you will find:

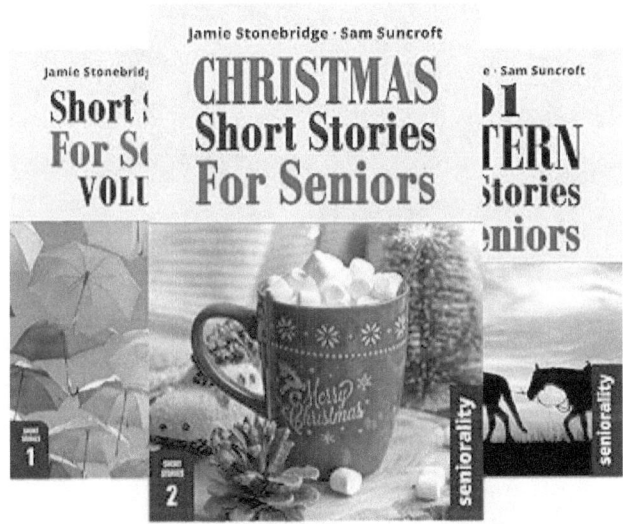

Short Stories

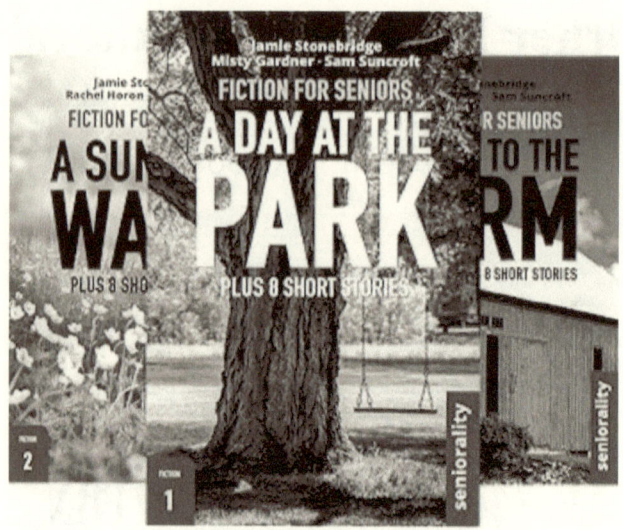

Fiction for Seniors

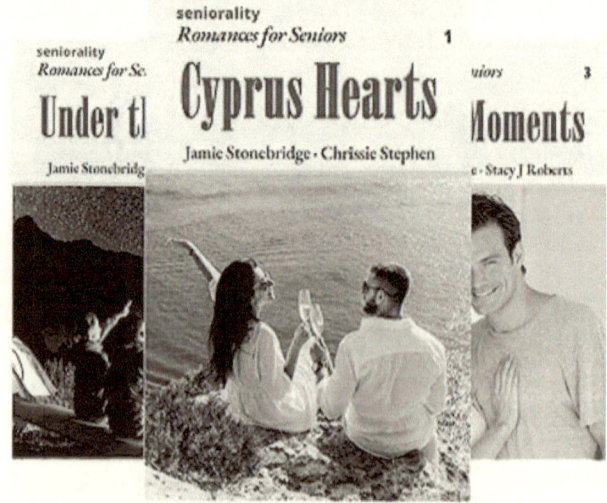

Romances for Seniors

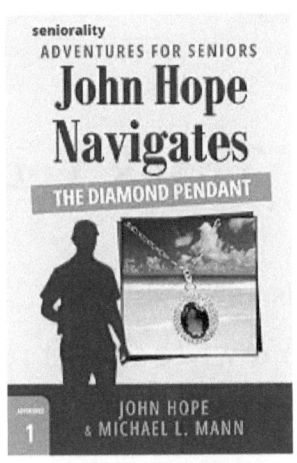

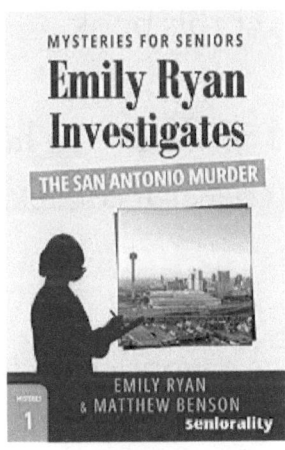

Find these books and many more
by searching on Amazon for
'seniorality'
or visit:

www.amazon.com/author/seniorality

Thank You

If you enjoyed this book or found it useful, we'd be very grateful if you'd write a short review on Amazon.

Your support really does make a difference and helps other people discover this book.

We personally read all reviews to hear how the books are being used, to collect feedback, and get ideas for future stories.

Thank you and have a wonderful day!

www.ingramcontent.com/pod-product-compliance
Lightning Source LLC
Chambersburg PA
CBHW020645220526
45464CB00001B/303